W0230523

Engineering
CHEMISTRY

Engineering
CHEMISTRY

FOR 3 YEAR DIPLOMA IN MECHANICAL ENGINEERING
[TECHNICIAN ENGINEERS EXAMINATION (PART I)]

Conducted by
INSTITUTION OF MECHANICAL ENGINEERS (INDIA)

Dr. S.P. Bakshi
M.Sc. Ph.D. (LONDON)
Retired Principal M.A.M. Govt. College,
Jammu Tawi.
Now Professor and Head of the Deptt.
of Chemistry, Jammu and Kashmir Institute
of Engineering Technology and Research, Kacchi Chowni,
Jammu Tawi.

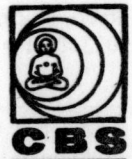

CBS Publishers & Distributors Pvt. Ltd.
New Delhi • Bengaluru • Chennai • Kochi • Kolkata • Mumbai
Hyderabad • Nagpur • Patna • Pune • Vijayawada

ISBN: 978-81-239-0134-3

First Edition: 1997
Reprint: 2003, 2017, 2019

Copyright © Publisher

All rights reserved. No part of this book may be reproduced or transmitted in any form or by any means, electronic or mechanical, including photocopying, recording, or any information storage and retrieval system without permission, in writing, from the publisher.

Published by **Satish Kumar Jain** and produced by **Varun Jain** for
CBS Publishers & Distributors Pvt. Ltd.,
4819/XI Prahlad Street, 24 Ansari Road, Daryaganj, New Delhi - 110002
delhi@cbspd.com, cbspubs@airtelmail.in • www.cbspd.com
Ph.: 23289259, 23266861, 23266867 • Fax: 011-23243014

Corporate Office: 204 FIE, Industrial Area, Patparganj, Delhi - 110 092
Ph: 49344934 • Fax: 011-49344935
E-mail: publishing@cbspd.com • publicity@cbspd.com

Branches:
• *Bengaluru:* 2975, 17th Cross, K.R. Road, Bansankari 2nd Stage,
  Bengaluru - 70 • Ph: +91-80-26771678/79 • Fax: +91-80-26771680
  E-mail: cbsbng@gmail.com, bangalore@cbspd.com
• *Chennai:* No. 7, Subbaraya Street, Shenoy Nagar, Chennai - 600030
  Ph: +91-44-26681266, 26680620 • Fax: +91-44-42032115
  E-mail: chennai@cbspd.com
• *Kochi:* Ashana House, 39/1904, A.M. Thomas Road, Valanjambalam,
  Ernakulum, Kochi • Ph: +91-484-4059061-65
  Fax: +91-484-4059065 • E-mail: cochin@cbspd.com
• *Kolkata:* 6-B, Ground Floor, Rameshwar Shaw Road, Kolkata - 700014
  Ph: +91-33-22891126/7/8 • E-mail: kolkata@cbspd.com
• *Mumbai:* 83-C, Dr. E. Moses Road, Worli, Mumbai - 400018
  Ph: +91-9833017933, 022-24902340/41 • E-mail: mumbai@cbspd.com

Representatives:

• Hyderabad: 0-9885175004	• Nagpur: 0-9021734563
• Patna: 0-9334159340	• Pune: 0-9623451994
• Jharkhand: 0-9811541605	• Uttarakhand: 0-9716462459

Printed at:
J.S. Offset Printers, Delhi (India)

Dedicated to
Late Professor E.E. TURNER
F.R.S.
Professor of Chemistry, London University,
London. An International Authority in
Stereo-Chemistry.

Preface to the First Edition

While teaching chemistry to Ist year students in the Jammu and Kashmir Institute of Engineering, Technology and Research, Jammu appearing in the 3 year Mech. Diploma of IME (Ind.) Examination. I have noted that no book in chemistry in the market covers the syllabus of Diploma of IME (Ind.) Examination. I have therefore written this book to meet the syllabus for the above Examination in its entirety. I have also written on topics which though not in the syllabus but have been asked in the Question Papers, to make the book more useful. The exercises at the and contains a large number of questions; some of which have been asked in this examination. I am greatful to authors from whose publications on the subject I have taken help in writing this book. I hope the present book will meet the demands of the students. Suggestions for improvement of the book will be received with thanks.

S.P. BAKSHI

About the Author

Teaching Chemistry for the last 45 years. Passed B.Sc. from Punjab University, Lahore in 1940, M.Sc. from Lucknow University, Lucknow in 1943 and Ph.D from London University, London in 1959. Worked with Professor E.E. Turner FRS. Published two papers in the journal of the Chemical Society, London in January, 1961, pages 168-170 and January 1961, pages 171-173.

Was a Professor and Head of the Department of Chemistry A.S. Govt. College, Srinagar and G.G.M. Science, College Jammu. Retired as Principal M.A.M. Govt. College, Jammu. Now Professor and Head of the Department of Chemistry, Jammu and Kashmir Institute of Engineering Technology and Research, Jammu

Have been a Paper Setter and Head Examiner in Chemistry of the B.Sc. Examination of the Jammu University, Jammu and J&K Board of School Education, Jammu for a number of years.

SYLLABUS
Engineering Chemistry
3 year Mech. Diploma of IME (India)

LAWS OF CHEMICAL COMBINATION: Law of Conservation of Mass, Law of Definite proportions, Law of Multiple proportions, Law of Reciprocal proportions, Explanation of the Laws of chemical combination in the light of Dalton's Atomic Theory.

THE KINETIC MOLECULAR THEORY: The main assumption of the theory, Kinetic equation for gases, $pv = \frac{1}{3} nmc^2$, and The Ideal Gas Law $pv = nRT$.

(Derivation of the equations not expected). Explanation of the gas laws by the Kinetic molecular theory, Boyle's Law, Charle's Law, Dalton's Law of partial pressures, Graham's Law of diffusion.

THE MOLE CONCEPT: Gay Lussac's Law of Combining Volumes, Avogadro's Law, Atomic Weights of Elements, Defination, determination, Determination of Atomic Weight using Dulong and Petit's Law, Molecular weight, Equivalent weight Defination, Relation between Equivalent weight, Atomic weight and Valency, Avogadro Number and the Mole, Weight and Volume relationship of gases.

ELECTRONIC STRUCTURE OF ATOM: Bohr's Theory of hydrogen Atom, Radius of Bohr orbit, Origin of spectral lines, Quantum theory.

PERIODICITY OF ELEMENTS:- Long form of the Periodic table and classification of Elements on the basis of electronic configurations, Trends of properties like valency, oxidation number, Atomic size, etc.

OSMOSIS AND OSMOTIC PRESSURE: Semipermeable membrane, Phenomenon of Osmosis, Osmotic pressure, Measurement of Osmotic pressure.

COLLOIDS: The Colloidal state of matter, Preparation of colloids, Mechanical, Electrical and Optical properties of Colloids, Coagulation of Colloids.

PRINCIPLES & METHODS OF PURIFICATION OF SUBSTAN-CES:- Crystalline and Amorphous Substances, Criteria of purity, Melting point and Boiling point as criteria of purity. Crystal-lisation-Fractional crystallisation, Purification of liquids. Distilla-tion, Fractional Distillation under reduced pressure.

FUELS: Classification of fuels and their chemical compositions. Characteristics of a good fuel, Calorific values. Solid Fuels-Coal, Types, Analysis of coal, lignite and peat. Liquid Fuels-Petroleum, Kerosene, Alcohol and their characterstics. Gaseous Fuels-Butane, Methane, Water Gas, Producer Gas, Coal Gas and its use in I.C. Engines, Marsh Gas. Nuclear-Plutonium, Uranium.

LUBRICANTS: Definition, Types of lubrication (Fluid film lubrica-tion and extreme Pressure lubrication), Classification of lubricants (Solid, Semi-solid, Liquid), Characteristics of lubricants (viscosity, viscosity index, oiliness, acidity, emulsification, flash and fire point, volatility, pour point, saponification value, Selection of lubricants for different types of Machinery.

ORES AND MINERALS: Minerals dressing general principles of concemtration of ores (Froth flotation, magnetic seperation and washing) Application of the electricity in the extraction of metals (Al, Zn) and refining of metals (Al, Zn and Cu).

METALLURGY OF IRON AND STEEL: Iron ores and minerals, chemistry of smelting of iron ores, acidic and basic fluxes, manufac-ture of pig-iron in blast furnace, cast iron and wrought iron manufacture, properties and uses.

Contents

Contents

Chapter I

Laws of Chemical Combination

There are five laws of Chemical Combination. They are:-

i) The law of conservation of mass;

ii) The law of constant composition or Definite proportion;

iii) The law of Multiple proportions;

iv) The law of Reciprocal Proportions;

v) The law of Gaseous Volumes (this is discussed in chapter III as per syllabus).

The first four refer to mass and the last one to gaseous volumes.

i) *LAW OF CONSERVATION OF MASS* (Lomonossoff, 1756). The Law of conservation of Mass states that matter can neither be created nor destroyed by any means or when a chemical change occurs, the total mass of the products is the same as the total mass of the reacting substances.

The truth of the law was exhaustively tested by Landolt 1900-1908. To mention, he studied the following two reactions in H-tube (Fig. 1.1)

i) Silver nitrate and potassium chromate solution giving a precipitate of silver chromate.

$$2\ AgNo_3 + K_2CrO_4 \longrightarrow 2\ KNO_3 + Ag_2CrO_4 \downarrow$$

ii) Silver Sulphate and ferrous sulphate giving precipitate of metallic silver.

$$Ag_2\ SO_4 + 2\ FeSO_4 \longrightarrow 2\ Ag \downarrow + Fe_2\ (SO_4)\ 3$$

One of the solutions was placed in one limb and the other in the second. It was sealed and weighed. On inverting the apparatus, the two solutions got mixed and reaction took

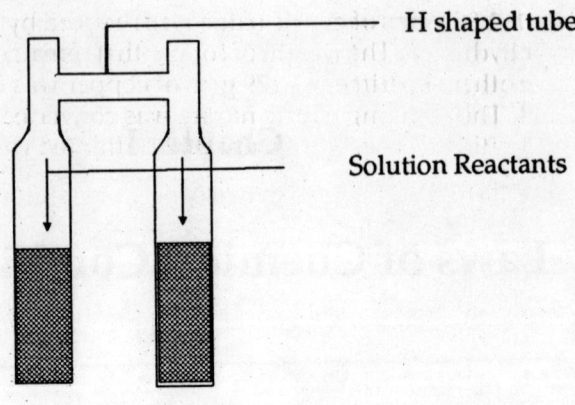

H shaped tube

Solution Reactants

Fig. 1.1: Landolt, Apparatus

place. After cooling and allowing to stand for sometime it was reweighed, it was found that the weight in each case remained unchanged.

iii) *LAW OF CONSTANT COMPOSITION OR DEFINITE PROPORTION, (PROUST, 1799).*
This law states that a chemical compound always consists of the same elements combined together in the same fixed proportion by weight.

As an example we take the case of Carbon dioxide. This can be prepared by:-

a) burning carbon

$$C + O_2 \underline{\hspace{2cm}} CO_2$$

b) by heating calcium carbonate

$$CaCO_3 \underline{\hspace{2cm}} CaO + CO_2$$

c) by heating Sodium bicarbonate

$$2NaHCO_3 \underline{\hspace{2cm}} Na_2CO_3 + CO_2 + H_2O$$

d) by the action of hydrochloric acid on sodium carbonate

$$Na_2CO_3 + 2HCl \underline{\hspace{2cm}} 2NaCl + H_2O + CO_2$$

Now if all these samples of carbon dioxide are analysied, it will be found that they contain carbon and oxygen combined together in the ratio of 12 gms of carbon and 32 gms of oxygen.

Example 1: 1.375 gms of cupric oxide was reduced by heating in a current of hydrogen. The weight of copper that remained was 1.098 gms. In another experiment 1.179 gms of copper was dissolved in nitric acid. The resulting cupric nitrate was converted into cupric oxide by ignition. The weight of cupric oxide formed was 1.476 gms.

Show that the results obtained in two experiments illustrate the law of constant composition.

Ist Experiment

wt. of copper in 1.375 gms of the oxide $\quad$ = 1.098 gms

$\therefore$ % of " in the compound = $\dfrac{1.098}{1.375} \times 100$ $\quad$ = 79.86%

2nd Experiment

Wt. of copper in 1.476 gms of oxide $\quad$ = 1.179 gms

$\therefore$ % of " in the oxide = $\dfrac{1.179}{1.1476} \times 100$ $\quad$ = 79.81%

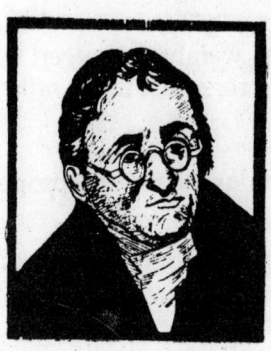

John Dalton (1776-1844)

Teacher, New College Manchester. Is regarded as one of the founders of modern Chemistry. He enunciated the Atomic Theory, the Law of Partial Pressures, the Law of Multiple Proportion and also devised a method of symbolising the elements and compounds.

Hence, we see that the percentage of copper and therefore, also of oxygen in the two samples of cupric oxide obtained by two different methods is practically the same. The results obtained, therefore, illustrate the law of constant composition.

iii) *LAW OF MULTIPLE PROPORTIONS (Dalton, 1803)*
The law of multiple proportions states that:-

When two elements combine to form two or more compounds, the weight of one element which combines with a fixed weight of the other, bear a simple ratio to one another.

Carbon combines with Oxygen to form two different compounds, carbon monoxide and carbon dioxide.

	Composition by weight	
	Carbon	*Oxygen*
Carbon Monoxide (CO)	12	16
Carbon Dioxide (CO_2)	12	32

The proportion of Oxygen combining with a constant weight 12 of carbon is 16 : 32 or 1 : 2.

Nitrogen forms as many as five stable oxides.

	Composition by weight	
	Nitrogen	*Oxygen*
Nitrous oxide N_2O	28	16×1
Nitric oxide NO	28	16×2
Nitrogen trioxide N_2O_3	28	16×3
Nitrogen tetra-oxide N_2O_4	28	16×4
Nitrogen penta-oxide N_2O_5	28	16×5

It is clear from the above figures that the weight of oxygen that combines with a fixed weight, 28 gms of nitrogen are in the ratio of

$$1 : 2 : 3 : 4 : 5$$

The two examples given above illustrate the law of multiple proportion.

Example 2: An element forms two oxides, one containing 53.33% and the other 36.36% of Oxygen. Show that these figures are in agreement with the law of Multiple proportions.

The percentage Composition of the two oxides are:

	% of Oxygen	% of element
First Oxide	53.33	100-53.33 = 46.67
Second Oxide	36.36	100-36.36 = 63.64

Hence, parts by weight of Oxygen in combination with 100 parts by weight of the given element in the two cases are:-

$$= \frac{53.33}{46.67} \times 100 = 114.5 \text{ parts}$$

$$= \frac{36.36}{63.64} \times 100 = 57.1 \text{ parts}$$

∴ The ratio of the weights of Oxygen that combines with a fixed weight (i.e., 100 parts) of the given element

$$= 114.5 : 57.1 \text{ or } 2 : 1$$

iv) *LAW OF RECIPROCAL PROPORTIONS (Richter, 1792)*
When two different elements unite with the same quantity of a third element the proportions in which they combine will be the same or a simple multiple of the proportions in which they unite with each other.

If W_1 gms of an element A combines with W_2 gms of another element B and also with W_3 gms of a third element C, then if the element B and C were to combine together they will do so in the ratio of $W_2 : W_3$ or a simple multiple there of.

Illustration

Take the case of Sulphus, Hydrogen and Oxygen.

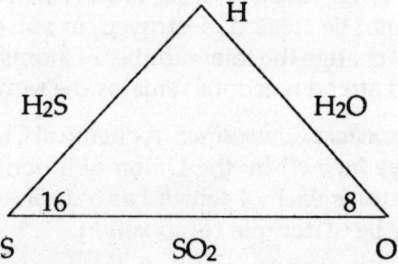

1 gm of hydrogen combines with 16.0 gms of Sulphur to form H_2S and 1.00 gms of hydrogen combines with 8 gms of Oxygen to form water. Therefore, if oxygen and sulphur combine they would do so in the proportion of 8/16. But Oxygen and Sulphur combine to form Sulphur Dioxide in the proportion of 1 gm of oxygen to 1.00 gms of sulphur. And we find te ratio 8/16 is simply related to the ratio 1/1 i.e., 1 : 2.

Example 3

Illustrate the Law of Reciprocal Proportions from the following data: Potassium chloride contains 52.5% Potassium. Potassium Iodide contains 23.6% potassium and Iodine Chloride contains 78.2% Iodine.

In KCl 52.5 gms of Potassium Combines with

47.5 gms of Chlorine.
In KI, 23.6 gms potassium combine with
76.4 gms of Iodine.
∴ in KI 52.5 gms of Potassium combines with

$$\frac{76.4}{23.6} \times 52.5 \text{ gms Iodine}$$

$$= 165.9 \text{ gms Iodine}$$

The ratio of the weights of Chlorine and Iodine which combine with the same weight of Potassium (viz., 52.5 gms) is $\frac{47.5}{165.9} = \frac{0.28}{1}$

Now in Iodine Chloride 78.2 gms of Iodine combines with 21.8 gms of chlorine.

$\therefore$ the ratio of the weights of chlorine and Iodine in the compound is $\frac{21.8}{78.2} = \frac{0.28}{1}$ this is related to the ratio found above as 1 : 1. This illustrates the law of Reciprocal Proportion.

Explanation of the laws of Chemical Combination by weight in the light of Dalton's Atomic theory.

i) *The law of conservation of Mass.* Since, according to Dalton, atoms cannot be created, destroyed, or sub divided during a chemical change the total number of atoms and their mass before and after a reactions remains the same.

ii) *The law of constant Composition.* A chemical Compound, since it is always formed by the Union of a definite number of different atoms each of which has a definite weight, must essentially be of definite composition.

iii) *The Law of Multiple Proportion.* If two elements combine to form more than one compound, let the formula of these compounds be AB_1, AB_2, AB_3 etc. Now if a and b are the atomic weights of A and B respectively the weights of the molecules of the Compound would be

a + 1b
a + 2b
a + 3b

It is clear that the weights, 1b, 2b, 3b of element B which combine with a constant weight a of A bear a ratio 1 : 2 : 3.

iv) *The Law of Reciprocal Proportion*
Let A, B and C represent three elements with atomic weights a, b and c respectively.
Now suppose

A + B ⟶ AB

A + C ⟶ AC

If B and C combine together, then atoms being indivisible, the resulting compound molecule will consist of either

> 1 atom of B + 1 atom of C
> or 1 atom of B + 2 atom of C
> or 1 atom of B + 3 atom of C, etc.

In these cases, the ratio of the weights of B and C which combine would be c/b, 2c/b, 3c/b etc., Thus, the proportion by weight in which B and C combine together must be simply related to the ratio c/b of weights of C and B which combine with a constant weight a of A. This is the law of reciprocal proportions

QUESTIONS

Law of Chemical Combination

1. State laws of chemical combination by weight.
   Illustrate your answer by examples.
   (U.P. Board 1944, 48, 53)
2. State the law of multiple proportions.
   Explain the law giving two examples.
3. State the law of Reciprocal proportions.
   Give suitable examples. (W-1988)

Law of Constant Composition.

4. The weight of Copper oxide obtained by treating 1.59 gms of metallic copper with concenterated HNO_3 and subsquent ignition was 1.99 gms. In another experiment, the weight of metallic copper produced by passing a current of hydrogen over 2.12 gms of heated copper oxide was found to be 1.694 gms. Show clearly that these figures are in accordance with the law of constant proportion.

5. Common salt obtained from a salt mine contained 60-67% of chlorine while 0.40 gms of a sample of common salt obtained from sea water contained 0.243 gms chlorine. Are these figures in accordance with the law of constant composition.

Law of Multiple Proportions.

6. A metal forms two oxides one of the oxide contains 77.78% Oxygen and the other 70.00% of the metal. Show that these results are in agreement with the Law of multiple proportions. (IIT Admission Test)

7. Manganese and Oygen form three compounds in which the percentage of Oxygen is 22.6, 36.9 and 50.6 respectively. Show that this is in accordance with the law of multiple proportions.   (Osmania Inter. 1954)

8. Two compounds each containing only tin and oxygen had the following composition.

Compound	% of Tin
A	78.77
B	88.12

Show that these data illustrate the law of multiple proportions.
(W-1988)

9. State the Law of multiple proportions and explain how for it applies to the different oxides of nitrogen.

(Delhi Prep. 1958)

Law of Reciprocal Proportions

10. The compounds CH_4, CO and H_2O contain the following percentages.

CH_4 : Carbon = 75% and Hydrogen = 25%
CO : Carbon = 42.86% and Oxygen = 57.14%
H_2O : Hydrogen = 11.11% and Oxygen = 88.89%

Show that they agree with the Law of reciprocal proportions.

11. PCl_3 contains 22.533% of Phosphorous and 77.46% chlorine, PH_3 contains 91.10% of Phosphorous, and 8.895% of hydrogen, HCl contains 2.764% of hydrogen and 97.235% of chlorine. Show that these data illustrate the Law of reciprocal proportions.

12. If a certain oxide of nitrogen weighing 11, g, yields 5.6 litres, of nitrogen and another oxide of nitrogen weighing 15 g also yields the same volume of nitrogen (all measurements being made at S.T.P) Show that the data cited supports the Law of multiple proportions.

13. From the following analysis of three compounds A,B and C, show that the Law of reciprocal proportions is illustrated:-

A = Carbon 14.47 %   Chlorine = 85.53%
B = Carbon 15.79%   Sulphur = 84.21%
C = Sulphur 47.44%   Chlorine = 52.56%

OBJECTIVE TYPE QUESTIONS

14.   *Fill in the blanks*

   i) The shorthand notation used for an element is called its
      _____   (S-1989)

   ii) Matter can be ————— created ————— destroyed.
                                                      (S-1989)

   iii) Atoms of the same elements with different atomic weights
        are called —————.

   iv) Atoms of the different elements with same atomic weights
       are called —————.

   v) The number of atoms present in a molecule of a gas is called
      —————.   (S-1989)

15. Choose the correct alternative from those given in each
        statement.   (W-1988)

   i) Properties of a compound are same/different from the
      properties of its elements.

   ii) A Physical change is a temporary/permanent change.

   iii) Glowing electric lamp is a physical/chemical change.

   iv) A chemical reaction is re-arrangement of atoms/molecules.

   v) Gases react together in a simple ratio of weights/volumes.

16. When two different elements unite with the same quantity
        of a third element, the proportion in which they combine will
        be the same or a simple multiple of the proportions in which
        they unite with each other. The above statement is known as
        the law of

   i) Conservasation of mass.
   ii) Multiple proportions.
   iii) Reciprocal proportions.
   iv) none of the above.

ANSWERS

   5. Yes
   14. i) Symbol ii) Neither, nor iii) Isotopes iv) Isobars v)
       Atomicity.
   15. i) Different ii) Temporary iii) Physical iv) Atoms v)
       Volumes.
   16. iii)

Chapter II

The Kinetic Molecular Theory of Gases

Kinesis = motion

The main assumptions of the theory:

According to this theory-

1) Gases consists of a very large number of separate tiny particles called molecules. The actual volume of the molecules is negligible as compared to the total volume of the gas.

2) There is no forces of attraction between the molecules which are completely independent of each other.

3) The molecules are moving very fast in straight lines at random colliding with each other and with the walls of the container. The pressure exerted by a gas is due to hits of its molecules on the walls of the container.

4) The molecules are perfectly elastic. Hence, there is no loss of kinetic energy resulting from their collisions or mutual friction.

5) The effect of gravity on the motion of the molecules is negligible in comparison to the effect of continued collisions between them.

6) The average kinetic energy of the gas molecules is directly proportional to the absolute temperature of the gas.

Kinetic equation for gases $PV = 1/3 \, nmv^2$,
where the total number of molecules is $= n$

the mass of one molecule is $= m$

and the root mean square velocity is $= v$
The ideal gas equation or the ideal gas law equation

$$PV = nRT$$

for one mole, this equation becomes $PV = RT$

(As per syllabus derivation of the equation is not expected)

Explanation of the gas laws by the kinetic molecular theory

a) Boyle's law: Temperature remaining constant the product of pressure and volume of a given mass of gas is constant. This law can be derived from the kinetic equation, $PV = 1/3\, nmv^2$ as follows:

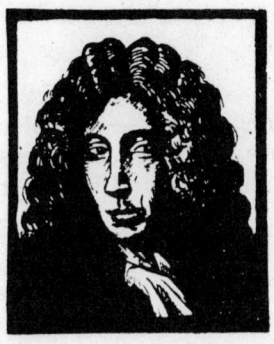

Rober Boyle (1627-91)

An Irish by birth, he was the greatest Scientist of England of his time.

It may be written as $PV = 2/3 \times 1/2\, nmv^2$ ... (i)

According to the kinetic theory, average kinetic energy is directly proportional to absolute temperature

i.e, $1/2\, nmv^2 \propto T$

or $1/2\, nmv^2 = KT$

Substituting this value in (i), we get

$$PV = 2/3\, KT$$

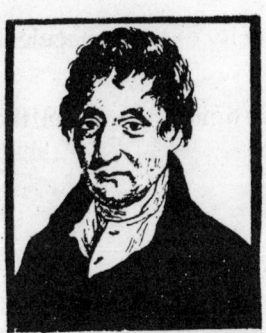

Jacques Alexandre Cesar Charles

(1746-1823)

A French Scientist of great repute, he was the first to make a balloon ascension with hydrogen and is known for his work on the effect of temperature on the volume of gases.

The product PV, therefore, will have a constant value at a constant temperature.

(b) *Charles Law:* According to this law, at constant pressure the volume of gas is directly proportional to the absolute temperature.

As derived above,

$$PV = 2/3 \, KT$$

or $V = 2/3 \, K/P \times T$

At constnat pressure

$$V = KT$$

or $V \propto T$

(c) Dalton's law of partial pressures:- Suppose n_1 molecules, each of mass m_1 of a gas A are contained in a vessel of volume V. Then, according to kinetic theory $PV = 1/3 \, nmv^2$

then pressure Pa of the gas will be given by

$$Pa = \frac{n_1 m_1 v_1^2}{3V}$$

Where V_1 is the root mean square velocity of the molecules of the gas A.

Now, suppose, n_2 molecules, each of mass m_2 of another gas B, are contained in the same vessel at the same temperature and there is no other gas present at that time. The pressure of this gas will be given by

$$Pb = \frac{n_2 m_2 v_2^2}{3v}$$

Where V_2 is the root mean square velocity of the molecules of the gas B.

If both the gases are present at the same time in the vessel, the total pressure p will be given by

$$P = \frac{n_1 m_1 v_1^2}{3V} + \frac{n_2 m_2 v_2^2}{3V} .$$

$$= pa + pb$$

Similarly, if three, four or more gases were present, the total pressure p will be given by

$$p = pa + pb + pc + pd + \ldots .$$

This is Dalton's Law of Partial pressures

Diffusion of Gases:- The property of gases by virtue of which they intermix with each other irrespective of the law of gravitation is known as Diffusion of gases.

Illustration- If a cylinder full of hydrogen is inverted over another cylinder full of bromine, it will be found after some time that the hydrogen has travelled from the upper to the lower cylinder and bromine has gone to the upper cylinder where it is conspicuous by its brown colour. These changes take place in direct contravention to the law of gravitation, the lighter hydrogen moving downward and the heavier bromine moving upwards.

Grahams Law of Diffusion of Gases: This law can be stated as follows:

Under similar conditions of temperature and pressure, the rates of diffusion of gases are inversely proportional to the square roots of their densities.

If r_1 and r_2 represent the rates of diffusion of two gases and d_1 and d_2 their respective densities, then

$$\frac{r_1}{r_2} = \sqrt{\frac{d_2}{d_1}}$$

Example: The rates of diffusion of ozone and carbon dioxide were found to be 27 and 28 respectively. The density of carbon dioxide is 22, find that of ozone.

$$\frac{r_1}{r_2} = \sqrt{\frac{d_2}{d_1}}$$

substituting Values,

$$\frac{27}{28} = \sqrt{\frac{22}{d_1}}$$

$$\therefore \frac{(27)^2}{(28)^2} = \frac{22}{d_1}$$

$$\therefore d_1 = \frac{28 \times 28 \times 22}{27 \times 27} = 23.7$$

Derivation of Grahams law of Diffusion of Gases:
$PV = 1/3 \, nmv^2$ Kinetic equation

$= 1/3 \, Mv^2$, where M is the total mass of the gas.

$$\therefore v^2 = \frac{3PV}{M}$$

$$= \frac{3P}{D} \text{ (where } D = M/V, \text{ the density of the gas)}$$

$$\text{or } V = \sqrt{\frac{3P}{D}}$$

Now, r the rate of diffusion of a gas is proportional to the root mean square velocity of its molecules i.e, $r \propto v$

Thus, we have $r \propto \sqrt{\frac{3P}{D}}$

$$\text{or } r \propto \sqrt{\frac{T}{D}}$$

if p is kept constant

or in other words, the rate of diffusion of a gas is inversely proportional to the square root of its density if the pressure remains constant. This is Graham's law.

QUESTIONS

1. State the main assumptions of the Kinetic Theory of gases. Deduce Boyle's law from Kinetic equation.

2. State the fundamental assumption of the Kinetic theory of gases. Deduce Graham's law of Diffusion from Kinetic equation.

3. State the postulates of the kinetic theory of gases and write the kinetic equation. Derive Charles law from it.

4. Give the postulates of the Kinetic theroy of gases and derive the laws of Boyle and Graham from the equation $PV = 1/3 \ nmv^2$.

5. The rates of diffusion of carbon dioxide and ozone were found to be 0.290 and 0.271 respectively. The density of CO_2 is 22. Find that of ozone. (S, 1989).

6. State and derive the Grahams law of diffusion. (W, 1989)

7. Describe in detail what do you know about "Diffusion phenomenon" (W, 1989)

OBJECTIVE TYPE QUESTIONS

8. *Fill in the blanks*

   1) The intermixing of two or more gases is called -----------. (S, 1989)

2) Gravity has-------- effect on the motion of gas molecules.

3) Average kinetic energy of a gas molecule is ---------- to absolute temperature.

4) According to kinetic theory of gases, a gas consist of discrete particles is called -----------

5) The theory dealing with the motion of molecules of gases is known as --------

ANSWERS

5. 25.19

8. (i) Diffusion (2) No (3) Directly proportional (4) Molecules (5) kinetic theory of gases.

Chapter III

The Mole Concept

Gay Lussac's Law of combining Volumes (1808)

The law may be stated as under:

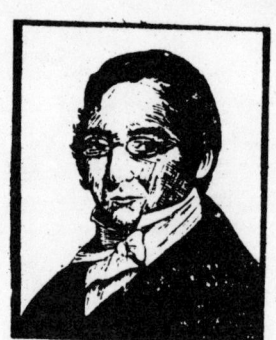

"When gases react together, they do so in volumes which bear a simples ratio to one another and to the volumes of the products, if these are gases, all measurements being made under the same conditions of temperature and pressure".

Joseph Louis Gay Lussac (1778-1854)

Was Professor of Chemistry at Ecole Polytechnique, France and Sorbonne University.

This law is illustrated by the following examples:

(1) One volume of nitrogen combines with three volumes of hydrogen to form two volumes of ammonia

$$N_2 \quad + \quad 3H_2 \longrightarrow 2\,NH_3$$

1 vol   3 vols   2 vols

(2) 2 volumes of sulphur dioxide combine with 1 volume of oxygen to form 2 volumes of sulphur trioxide

$$2\,SO_2 \quad + \quad O_2 \longrightarrow 2\,SO_3$$

2 vols   1 vol   2 vols

(3) 1 volume of hydrgen combine with 1 volume of chlorine to form 2 volumes of hydrochloric acid

$$H_2 \quad + \quad Cl_2 \longrightarrow 2HCl$$

1 vol   1 vol   2 vols

(4) Two volumes of hydrgen combine with 1 volume of oxygen to form two volumes of steam

$$2 H_2 + O_2 \longrightarrow 2 H_2O$$
2 vols   1 vol   2 vols

(5) 1 volume of nitrogen combines with 1 volume of oxygen to form two volumes of nitric oxide

$$N_2 + O_2 \longrightarrow 2 NO$$
1 vol   1vol   2 vols

Avogadro's law

In 1811, Avogadro, an Italian chemist postulated the existence of two kinds of particles of which matter is made up:

i) Atom, the smallest particles of elements which take part in chemical changes; and

ii) Molecule is the particle of an element or compound which is capable of independent existence. A molecule of an element may contain one or more atoms but a molecule of a compound must necessarily contain at least two atoms. After making the above assumption he stated his hypothesis, which is now known as Avogadro's law as follows:

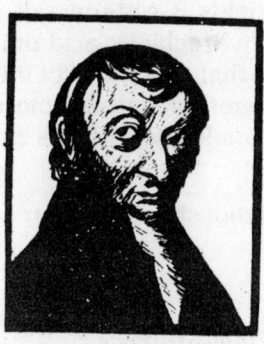

" Equal volumes of all gases, under similar conditions of temperature and pressure, contain the same number of molecules."

Amedeo Avogadro (1776-1856)

An Italian Scientist, he was Professor at Turin. He is famous for the hypothesis which bears his name.

Importance and usefulness of Avogadro's law

It may be summarised as under:

(1) It has put the atomic theory on a firm footing by making clear the distinction between atoms and molecules.

(2) Explanation of Gay lussac's law of Gaseous Volumes.

Taking the case of hydrogen-chlorine combination 1 volume of hydrogen + 1 volume of chlorine = 2 volumes of hydrochloric acid.

Applying Avogadro's law:

n molecules of hydrogen + n molecules of chlorine = 2 n molecules of hydrochloric acid.

It means one molecule of hydrochloric acid contains 1/2 molecule of hydrogen and 1/2 molecule of chlorine. Now, half a molecule of hydrogen or chlorine may consist of one or more atoms. Hence Gay-Lussac's law no longer conflicts with Dalton's Theory.

(3) Determination of Atomicity of Hydrogen and other elementary gases. Atomicity of an element is the number of atoms, present in its molecule.

In (2) above we have shown that one molecule of hydrochloric acid contains 1/2 molecule of hydrogen + 1/2 molecule of chlorine. Hence, it follows that a molecule of hydrogen must contain 2, 4, 6 or an even member of atoms.

The number of sodium salts that can be obtained from an acid depends on the replaceable hydrogen atoms present in its molecule.

H_2SO_4 ———————— $NaHSO_4$, Na_2SO_4 (2 salts)

H_3PO_4 ———————— NaH_2PO_4, Na_2HPO_4, Na_3PO_4 (3 salts)

Thus, sulphuric acid which yields two sodium salts has 2 hydrogen atoms and phosphoric acid which yields 3 sodium salt has 3 hydrogen atoms. Now, in the case of hydrochloric acid only one sodium salt is obtained which indicates that a molecule of this acid contains only one hydrogen atom. Therefore, half a molecule of hydrogen gas contains 1 atom, or one molecule contains 2 atoms i.e., hydrogen is diatomic.

(4) It has helped in deducing the relationship Molecular weight = 2 vapour density

or M.Wt.= 2 V.D.

$$V.D. = \frac{\text{Wt. of certain volume of the substance}}{\text{Wt. of the same volume of hydrogen}}$$

Applying Avogadro's Hypothesis, we have

$$V.D. = \frac{\text{Wt. of n molecules of the substance}}{\text{Wt. of n molecules of hydrogen}}$$

$$= \frac{\text{Wt. of 1 molecule of the substance}}{\text{Wt. of 1 molecule of hydrogen}} \qquad ...(i)$$

$$\text{Now, M.Wt.} = \frac{\text{Wt. of 1 molecule of the substance}}{\text{Wt. of 1 atom of hydrogen}} \qquad ...(ii)$$

Dividing (ii) by (i), we get

$$\frac{\text{M.Wt.}}{\text{V.D.}} = \frac{\text{Wt. 1 molecule of Hydrogen}}{\text{Wt. of 1 atom of Hydrogen}}$$

Since 1 molecule of hydrogen contains 2 atoms

$$\frac{\text{M.Wt.}}{\text{V.D.}} = 2 \text{ or M.Wt.} = 2 \text{ V.D.}$$

This relationship is very useful in the determination of molecular weights.

   (5) It gives a relationship between the volumes and weights of gases

22.4 litres of any gas at N.T.P. will contain its molecular weights in grams. It has been found experimentally that 22.4 litres of hydrogen at N.T.P. weigh equal to 2 grams i.e., its molecular weight in grams. According to Avogadro's law, equal volumes of all gases under the same conditions of temperature and pressure contain equal number of molecules and hence it follows that:

22.4 litres of any gas at N.T.P. will contain 1 gm. molecule or molecular weight in grams. This relation also helps us in the determination of molecular weight.

   (6) This law helps in the calculation of the molecular formulae of gases and is useful in Gas Analysis.

If the volumes of the reactant and the products are known, the molecular formula can be found out without further data.

For example:

1 vol of Nitrogen + 3 vols of Hydrogen → 2 vols of Ammonia

If n be the number of molecules in 1 vol according to Avogadro's law

n molecules of Nitrogen + 3 n molecules of hydrogen → 2n molecules of ammonia.

or 1 molecule of nitrogen + 3 molecules of hydrogen → 2 molecules of ammonia.

Since, Nitrogen and Hydrogen are diatomic, 2 atoms of Nitrogen + 6 atoms of Hydrogen → 2 molecules of ammonia

∴ 1 molecule of ammonia contains 1 atom of Nitrogen and 3 atoms of Hydrogen. Hence, the molecular formula of ammonia is NH_3.

   (7) It helps in the determination of atomic weights.

Atomic Weights of Elements:

Definition: The atomic weight of an element is defined as the average mass of its atom in atomic mass unit compared with the weight of carbon atom taken as 12 in atomic mass unit.

Determination of atomic weight by Dulong and Petit's Law

In 1818, two Frenchmen, Dulong and Petit, found that a close relation existed between the atomic weights and the specific heats of elements in the solid state and enunciated an emperical rule called Dulong and Petit's Law, which may be stated thus:

"The product of the atomic weight and the specific heat of an element in the solid state is approximately 6.4"

$$\text{or approximate atomic weight} = \frac{6.4}{\text{Specific heat}}$$

Exact atomic weight = Eq. wt. × valency

Example: 1

2.380 gm of tin, on treatment with conc. nitric acid and subsequent ignition, gave 3.022 gm of oxide. The specific heat of the metal is 0.055. Calculate the exact atomic weight of tin.

2.380 gm of tin combines with 3.022 - 2.380, or 0.642 gm of oxygen

$$\therefore \text{Eq. wt. of tin} = \frac{2.380 \times 8}{0.642} \text{ or } 29.66$$

By Dulong and Petit's law, the approximate atomic weight of tin

$$= \frac{6.4}{0.055} \text{ or } 116$$

Hence, Valency of tin $= \dfrac{116}{29.66}$ or 4 (to the nearest whole number)

Exact atomic wt. of tin = Eq. wt. × Valency
$$= 29.66 \times 4$$
$$= 118.6$$

Molecular Weight

Molecular weight of a substance (element or compound) is defined as the weight of one molecule of the substance as compared to the weight of carbon taken as 12.

The molecular weight of a substance is obtained by adding up the atomic weights of the constituent atoms present in one molecule of the substance.

Thus, molecular weight of $CaCO_3$:

$$(Ca = 40, C = 12, O = 16) = 40 + 12 + 48 = 100$$

The atomic and molecular weights when expressed in gms are termed as gram atom and gram molecule (or mole) respectively of the substance concerned.

Equivalent weight

The equivalent weight of a substance is the number of parts by weight of it which combine with or displace 8 parts by weight of oxygen or 1 parts by weight of hydrogen or 35.5 parts by weight of chlorine. The gram equivalent weight of a substance is the equivalent weight expressed in grams.

Determination of equivalent weight

Some of the common method employed for the determination of equivalent weight are described below:

(1) Hydrogen displacement method. Metal like iron, zinc and magnesium can displace hydrogen from acids and while metal like sodium, Potassium and calcium can displace hydrogen from water or alcohol. A small quantity of metal is accurately weighed and reacted with excess of acid. The volume of hydrogen evolved is measured and its weight calculated. (We know that 2 gms of hydrogen occupy 22.4 litres at S.T.P.)

(2) Oxide formation method-

(a) Direct oxidation. A weighed quantity of the element is converted into its oxide by heating it in a current of oxygen. After cooling the oxide is weighed and weight of the combined oxygen calculated. Then,

$$\frac{\text{Eq. Wt. of metal}}{\text{Eq. Wt. of oxygen}} = \frac{\text{Wt. of metal}}{\text{Wt. of oxygen}}$$

This method has been used for the determination of the equivalent weights of Mg, Carbon, Phosphorous.

(b) Indirect oxidation. Metals like Cu, Sn and Fe, which do not form oxides easily are dissolved in conc HNO_3 and nitrate thus formed is then decomposed into the oxide by ignition.

(3) Reduction of an oxide. A weighed quantity of the oxide is heated and reduced in a current of hydrogen. The weight of

the metal left behind is determined and the equivalent weight determined by finding the weight of the metal that combines with 8 parts by weight of oxygen.

(4) By combination with chlorine. In this method the equivalent weight is found by forming the chloride and calculating the weight of the element combining with 35.5 parts by weight of the chlorine.

(5) *Metal displacement method*

Copper is displaced from Copper Sulphate solution by the addition of iron. If the equivalent weight of iron is known that of Copper can be calculated by finding out the weight of Copper desposited and the weight of iron dissolved.

$$\frac{\text{Wt. of Copper}}{\text{Wt. of Iron}} = \frac{\text{Eq. Wt. of Copper}}{\text{Eq. Wt. of Iron}}$$

(6) By Double Decomposition. In the change $AB + CD \to AD + BC$, if we know the weights of AB and AD and the eq. wts. of A & D, the equivalent weight of B can be calculated from the relation.

$$\frac{\text{Wt. of AB}}{\text{Wt. of AD}} = \frac{\text{Eq. Wt. of A} + \text{Eq. Wt. of B}}{\text{Eq. Wt. of A} + \text{Eq. Wt. of D}}$$

(7) By electrolysis. According to Faraday's second law of electrolysis, if the same current is passed through solution of different electrolytes, the weights of different elements liberated at the electrodes are proportional to their Chemical equivalents.

The same current is passed for a given time through solution of salts of two metals e.g., copper sulphate and silver nitrate, connected in series. The increase in weight of cathode in each case gives the weight of the metal deposited knowing the weight of metals deposited and the equivalent wt. of one of these the equivalent wt. of the other metal can be calculated. The eq. wt. of copper is determined from the relation:

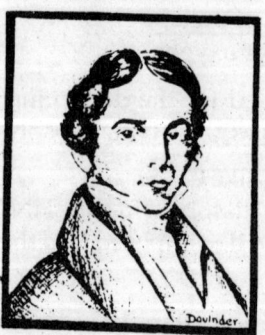

Michael Faraday (1791-1867)

An English Physicis and Chemist who is well known for his outstanding work on electrolysis.

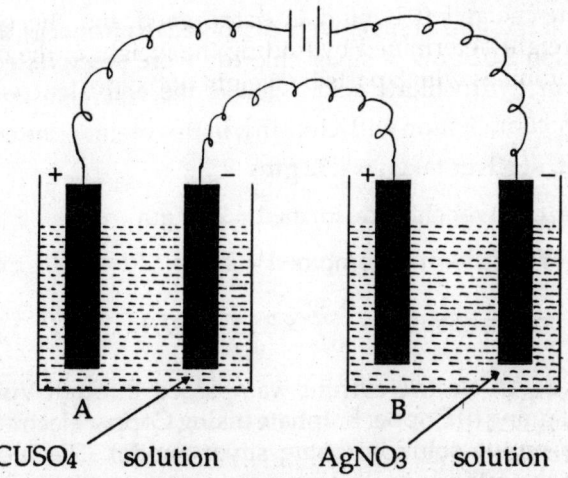

Fig. 3.1

$$\frac{\text{Wt. of Cu deposited}}{\text{Wt. of Ag deposited}} = \frac{\text{Eg. Wt. of Cu}}{\text{Eq. Wt. of Ag}}$$

Determination of equivalent weight by Electrolysis.

Example 2: 0.525 gm of metal on oxidation gave 0.75 gm of oxide. Calculate the equivalent weight of the metal.

Wt. of the metal = 0.525 gm

Wt. of the oxide = 0.75 gm

∴ Wt. of Oxygen = 0.225 gm

Hence, wt. of the metal combining with 8 gms of oxygen = $\frac{8 \times 0.525}{0.225}$ = 18.7 Ans.

Example 3: 0.79 gms of copper oxide, on heating in a current of hydrogen gave 0.63 gm of copper. Calculate the equivalent weight of copper.

wt. of copper oxide = 0.79 gm

wt. of copper formed = 0.63 gm

wt. of oxygen that combines with 0.63 gm of copper = 0.16

wt. of copper that combines with 8 gms of

oxygen = $\frac{8 \times 0.63}{0.16}$ = 31.5 gms

∴ Eq. wt. of Copper = 31.5

Example 4: 1.52 gms of silver were dissolved in nitric acid, and from this solution 2.02 gms of silver chloride were precipitated by the addition of hydrochloric acid. what is the equvalent weight of silver?

Wt. of silver taken = 1.52 gms

Wt. of silver chloride formed = 2.02 gm

∴ Wt. of chlorine combined = 2.02 – 1.52 = 0.50 gms

∴ Eq. wt. of silver = $\dfrac{1.52}{0.5} \times 35.5 = 107.9$

Example 5: An electric current was passed through Voltameter Cells containing (i) Copper Sulphate (using Copper electrodes) and (ii) Silver nitrate solution (using silver anode). The increase in weight of the cathode in the two cases was respectively 0.195 gm. and 0.661 gm. Calculate the Chemical equivalent of copper taking that of silver as 107.9

Wt. of copper deposited = 0.195 gm

Wt. of silver deposited = 0.661 gm

Eq. wt. of silver = 107.9

Therefore, $\dfrac{0.195}{0.661} = \dfrac{\text{Eq. wt. of Cu}}{107.9}$

∴ Eq. wt. of Cu. = $\dfrac{0.195 \times 107.9}{0.661} = 31.8$

Relation between equivalent weight, Atomic weight and Valency.

Atomic weight = Eq. wt. × Valency

Equivalent wt. = $\dfrac{\text{Atomic wt.}}{\text{Valency}}$

Valency $\dfrac{\text{Atomic Wt.}}{\text{Equivalent Wt.}}$

Avogadro Number and the Mole

A mole is the chemist unit for counting atoms, molecules, ions and other similar objects. A mole means a collection of 6.023×10^{23} particles. This value has been determined by a variety of methods. This number of particles is called Avogadro's Number and is represented by the symbol N.

1 mole = 6.023×10^{23} particles.

= Gram atomic mass in case of an atom

= Gram molecular mass in case of molecule

= 22.4 litres at S.T.P. in case of a gas

Example 6: How many atoms are there in 16 gms of oxygen – 16

Atomic mass of oxygen = 16 amu

Gram atomic mass of oxygen = 16 gm

No. of moles of oxygen = 16/16 = 1

No. of atoms in 1 mole of oxygen = 6.023×10^{23}

Example 7: Calculate the number of molecules in a drop of water weighing 0.05 gm (H = 1; O = 16)

Gram molecular mass of water = 18 gms

No. of molecules in 18 gms of water (1 mole of water) = 6.023×10^{23}

$\therefore$ No. of molecules in 0.05 gms of water

$$= \frac{6.023 \times 10^{23} \times 0.05}{18} = 1.673 \times 10^{21} \text{ molecules}$$

Weight and Volume relationship of gases

Avogadro's law has led to the deducation: 22.4 litres of any gas at S.T.P. will contain its molecular weight in grams.

It has been experimentally found that 22.4 litres of hydrogen at S.T.P. weigh equal to 2 grams, i.e., its molecular weight in grams. According to Avogadro's law, equal volumes of all gases under the same conditions of temperature and pressure contain equal number of molecules and hence it follows that:

22.4 litres of any gas at S.T.P. will contain 1 gram molecule or its molecular weight in grams. This relationship also helps us in the determination of molecular weight.

M. wt. being

Thus, the weight of 22.4 litres of oxygen at S.T.P. = 32   32

The weight of 22.4 litres of Carbon dioxide at S.T.P. = 44 gms   44

The weight of 22.4 litres of chlorine at S.T.P. = 71 gms   71

The molecular weight of a gas being known the weight of any volume of the gas under any conditions of temperature and pressure can be easily calculated.

Example 8: How many grams of sulphur dioxide will occupy a volume of 5.6 litres at S.T.P.

1 gram molecular weight of sulphur dioxide

$$SO_2 = 32 + 2 \times 16 = 64 \text{ gms}$$

Therefore, 22.4 lits of SO_2 at S.T.P. weigh 64 gms

∴ 5.6 lits of SO_2 will weigh $64/22.4 \times 5.6 = 16$ gms

Example 9: Determine the (i) weight and (ii) volume of carbon dioxide evolved at S.T.P. by heating 1 gm of calcium carbonate (At. wt. Ca = 40, C = 12, O = 16)

$$CaCO_3 \text{----------} CaO + CO_2$$

1 gm molecular wt.   1 gm molecular wt.

$40 + 12 + 48 = 100$ gm $12 + 32 = 44$ gm

100 gms of $CaCO_3$ when heated produce $CO_2 = 44$ gms

∴ 1 gm of $CaCO_3$ will produce $44/100 = 0.44$ gm CO_2.

1 gm mol. wt. of CO_2 = 22400 CC CO_2 at S.T.P.

∴ 44 gms of CO_2 = 22400 CC CO_2 at S.T.P.

1 gm -------- = 22400/44 —do—

0.44 ------- = $22400/44 \times 0.44$ CO_2 at S.T.P.

= 224 CC at S.T.P.

QUESTIONS

1. Explain giving examples, Gay Lussac's law of gaseous Volumes.   (S-1989), (S-1990)

2. Enunciate Avaogadro's law and show its importance in Chemistry.

3. Derive relationship between molecular wt. and the vapour density of a gas or Vapour with the help of Avogadro's hypothesis.   (S-1989)

4. Enunciate Avogadro's law and apply it to establish the atomicity of hydrogen.

5. a) Define atomic weight and molecular weight.

    b) Deduce the relation between equivalent weight and atomic weight.

    c) State Dulong and Petit's law.

6. How will you determine equivalent weight by different methods? Name them only. (W-1989)

7. What is meant by the terms atomic weight and equivalent weights. Describe any two methods for the determination of the equivalent weight of a metal. 0.5595 gm of a metal when changed into its chloride weighs 0.717 gm. The specific heat of the metal is 0.059 calories. What is the correct atomic weight of the metal? (Cl = 35.5)

8. a) Define equivalent weight of a metal.

    b) Derive the relationship between equivalent weights, atomic weight and valency?

9. An electric current is passed through solutions of copper sulphate and cyanide of silver connected in series. If in a given times 0.35 gm of copper is deposited. What will be weight of silver deposited in the same time.

    (At. wt. Cu = 63.57, Ag = 107.8

10. What is the number of moles in 10 gm of $CaCO_3$?

11. What do you understand by a Mole? Calculate the mass of an atom of silver.

12. What will be the volume of 8 gm of Oxygen at S.T.P. (S-1989)

13. What volume of CO_2 is produced at S.T.P. on burning 80 gm of charcoal?

14. 0.2 gm of pure metal on ignition gave 0.333 gm of its oxide What is the equivalent weight of metal?

15. 2.5 gms of magnesium when heated combine with 1.66 gm of Oxygen-Find the equivalent weight of magnesium. (W-1989)

16. a) Define gram equivalent weight.

    b) Describe givin g examples a method to determine equivalent weight.

    1 gm of chloride of a metal gave 0.203 gm of the metal.

Calculate equivalent weight of the metal.

At. wt of Cl_2 = 35.5 (W-1988)

17. a) Define and explain the following:

    i) Boyle's law   ii) Charles law.

    b) Derive general gas equation from Boyle's and Charles law's.

    c) Volume of gas collected over water at $13^\circ C$ measured 47.8 ml under pressure 765 mm. What would be the volume of dry gas at NTP? (Aqueous Tension at $13^\circ C$ = 11.2 mm.) (S-1988)

18. Calculate the volume which would be possessed by 15 gm of CO_2 gas at $15^\circ C$ and 720 mm pressure.

    (C = 12, O= 16 are the atomic weights) (S-1990)

19. An electric current was passed in series through dilute sulphuric acid and copper sulphate solution (using copper electrodes) evolved 110 cc of Hydrogen measured at $13^\circ c$ and 765 mm pressure and deposited 0.296 gm of copper Calculate equivalent of copper (Aqueous vapour pressure at $13^\circ C$ = 11 mm). (W-1989)

OBJECTIVE TYPE QUESTIONS

20. *Fill in the blanks*

    i) Pressure of dry gas = pressure of moist gas + ----------

    ii) The number of atoms present in a molecule of a gas is called ----------.

    iii) One gram molecule of every gas occupies ------ at ------.

    iv) Molecular weight = -----------× V.D. (S-1989)

21. Choose the correct alternative from those given in each statement: (W-1988)

    i) The number of replaceable hydrogen atoms in sulphric acid is one/two.

    ii) The volume of gas at – $273^\circ C$. Zero/hundred ml.

    iii) The smallest particle of a gas which can have free existance is called element/molecule.

iv) One gram molecule of every gas occupies 22.4/22400 litrs at NTP.

ANSWERS

(7) 126.1 (9) 1.19 gms (10) 0.1 mole (11) 1.79×10^{-22} gm (12) 5.6 litres (13) 149.33 litres. (14) 12.03 (15) 12.0 4 (16) (c) 9 .042 (17) (c) 45.25 ml (18) 8.05 litres (19) 31.48

(20) (i) Pressure of Water vapours (in place + put-), (ii) Atomicity (iii) 22.4 litres, STP., (iv) 2.

(21) (i) 2, (ii) Zero, (iii) molecule, (iv) 22.4 litres.

Chapter IV

Electronic Structure of Atom

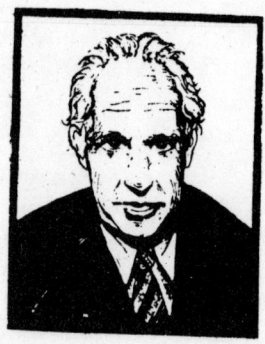

Neils Bohr (1885-

Danish Physicist; was awarded Nobel prize for Physics in 1922; greatly extended theory of atomic structure by devising an atomic model in 1913 and evolving theory of nuclear structure; assisted America in Atom Bomb research.

Failure of Rutherford's Atomic Model. According to Rutherford's atomic model, an atom consists of a nucleus and the electrons are revolving around it. Thus, the centrifugal force which is produced by the circulations of electrons balances the force of attraction between the electrons and the nucleus.

But Clark Maxwell had shown that a charged particle which move under the influence of a attractive force continuously lose energy. Since electron is also a charged particle, it must emit radiations and thus lose energy continuously. As the electron loses energy, it starts coming nearer the nucleus i.e., its orbit would become smaller and smaller. As a result of this, the electron would ultimately fall into the nucleus. But we know that the revolving electrons never fall into the nucleus. Thus, Rutherford's picture of an atom is faulty.

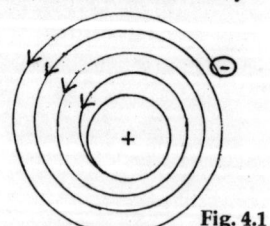

The orbit becoming smaller and smaller.

Fig. 4.1

Bohr's Atomic Model

To overcome the drawbacks in the Rutherford's atomic model, in 1913 Niel Bohr a Danish physicist proposed his model of the atom.

The following are the postulates of the Bohr's atomic model:

1. The electrons revolve round the nucleus in certain permitted circular orbits. These orbits are called energy shells or energy levels (K,L,M,N,....levels as they are associated with definite amounts of energies).

2. So long as the electron revolves in a particular orbit, it does not emit energy. It is due to this reason that the circular orbits are called stationary states or definite energy levels.

3. The orbits of allowed electronic motion are those in which the angular momentum of the electron is an integral multiple of $\dfrac{nh}{2\pi}$.

The angular momentum $mvr = \dfrac{nh}{2\pi}$

Where, m = mass of an electron

v = velocity of orbit

r = radius of orbit

n = number of the orbit and

h = Plank's constant = 6.62×10^{-27} erg.

4. Since the charge in energy takes place in quanta, an electron cannot enter gradually from one orbit to the other, it can only enter the other orbit by jumps.

    (a) When an electron jumps from higher orbit with energy E_2 to lower orbit with energy E_1, then the difference of energy is emitted as a radiation. It follows the relation:

    $E_2 - E_1 = h\gamma$

    (b) When an electron jumps from lower orbit with energy E_1 to higher orbit with energy E_2, then the difference of energy is absorbed. It follows the relation:

    $E_2 - E_1 = h\gamma$

Defects of Bohr's Model

Following are a few of the short comings of the Bohr's atomic model:

(i)   It explains fully the spectrum of hydrogen but could not explain the spectra and energy of polyelectron atoms (atoms having more than one electron).

(ii) It could not account for brightness of spectral lines.

(iii) According to Bohr, the circular orbits of the electrons are planar. However the modern researches show that an electron moves round the nucleus in three dimensional space (X, Y, Z - axis).

(iv) It could not explain why atoms combine to form molecules and the shape of the molecules.

(v)   One of the major drawbacks of Bohr's theory is that it assumes a definite knowledge about position and momentum of electrons at the same time.

However, Heisenberg (1927) suggested that it is impossible to measure simultaneously both the exact position and momentum of the subatomic particle such as electron. This statement is known as Heisenberg's Uncertainty Principle.

Bohr's theory as applied to hydrogen atom

Hydrogen has only one electron when this electron is knocked out by some method, the residue is hydrogen nucleus with a positive charge. This hydrogen nucleus has same power of attraction for the electron. Now let there be an electron lying at a certain distance from the nucleus. **The electron has some potential energy but** when the same electron comes into the orbit of the hydrogen nucleus, it will have less energy. The difference in the two energies will be radiated in the form of light. Since hydrogen atom has only one orbit, the energy so radiated will always be the same.

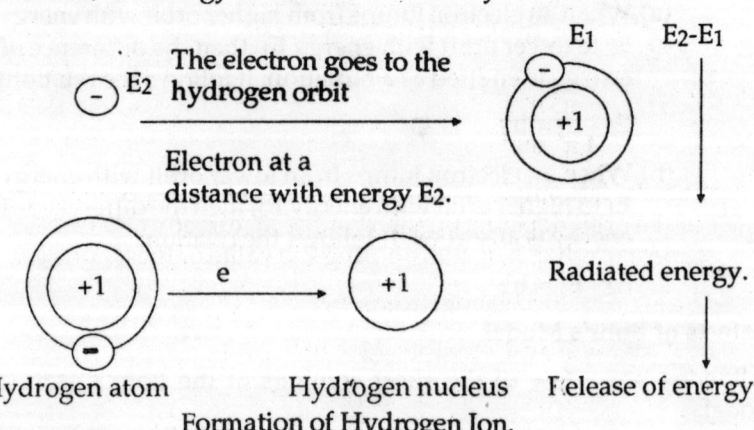

Hydrogen atom   Hydrogen nucleus   Release of energy

Formation of Hydrogen Ion.

Fig. 4.2

Radius of Bohr's orbit

The basis for the size of any orbit is that the electron moving in any of these orbits has centrifugal force equal to the force of attraction which the nucleus exerts on the revolving electron.

The centrifugal force with which an electron is moving in a circular path is equal to mass x acceleration, i.e., $F = ma$

But acceleration of the electron moving in an orbit of radius r and linear velocity 'v' is equal to $\dfrac{v^2}{r}$

$$\therefore F = m.\dfrac{v^2}{r}$$

According to Coulomb's law of force between two charges i.e., +e of the nucleus and -e of the electron lying at a distance r cms., the force of attraction will be $= \dfrac{e^2}{r^2}$

Thus, $\dfrac{mv^2}{r} = \dfrac{e^2}{r^2}$ or $r = \dfrac{e^2}{mv^2}$

from the equation of angular momentum.

$$mvr = n \times \dfrac{h}{2\pi}$$

$$v = \dfrac{n}{mr} \times \dfrac{h}{2\pi}$$

Substituting this value of the V in the equation,

$$\dfrac{mv^2}{r} = \dfrac{e^2}{r^2}, \text{ we have } r = \dfrac{e^2}{mv^2}$$

$$r = \dfrac{n^2 h^2}{4\pi^2 me^2}$$

When 'n' is a simple whole number integer i.e. 1, 2, 3, ... The radius r of the orbit depends on the value of 'n' directly and on the value of constants like h, π. Substituting the value of these constants.

$$r = n^2 (0.529) \text{ angstroms}$$

(One Angstrom unit $= 1 \times 10^{-8}$ cm)

Thus when n = 1, r = 1×0.529 Å

This is often considered to be the value of the radius of the hydrogen atom.

When $n = 2, r = (2)^2 \times 0.529 = 4 \times 0.529 = 2.116$ Å .

When $n = 3, r = (3)^2 \times 0.529 = 9 \times 0.529 = 4.761$ Å and so on.

Origin of Spectral Lines

Hydrogen has only on electron in its atom but any sample of hydrogen contains almost infinite number of atoms and hence electrons. When hydrogen gas is subjected to electric discharge taken in a discharge tube under low pressure, individual electrons present in its atoms (from molecule) absorb different quantities of energy, thus excited to different energy levels. The excited electrons then jump back to their original energy levels (ground states) giving rise to the emmission of radiations of different fre- quencies. Each electronic transition produçes spectral lines consist- ing of a few sharp lines and seperated by dark bands is called line spectrum.

Discharge Hydrogen tube

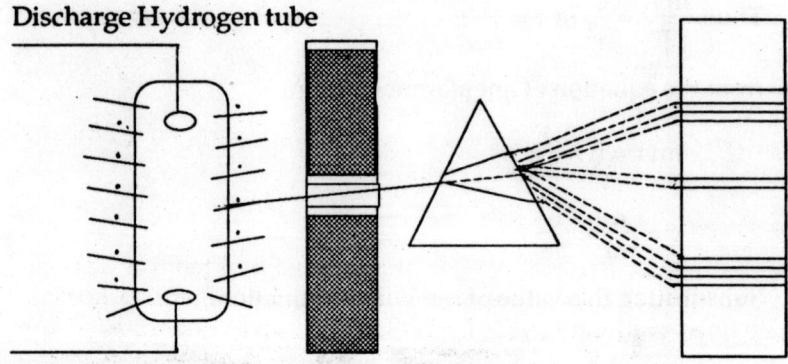

Fig. 4.3   Line spectrum of hydrogen

The lines costituting the hydrogen spectrum, resulting from electronic transitions involving eight energy levels, have been grouped into five series which are named after their discoverer and are given as under:

   (i)   Lyman series .... Ultra-Violet region
  (ii)   Balmar series .... Visible region
 (iii)   Paschen series .... Infra-Red region
  (iv)   Brackett series .... Infra-Red region and
   (v)   P fund series .... Infra-Red region.

Diagram

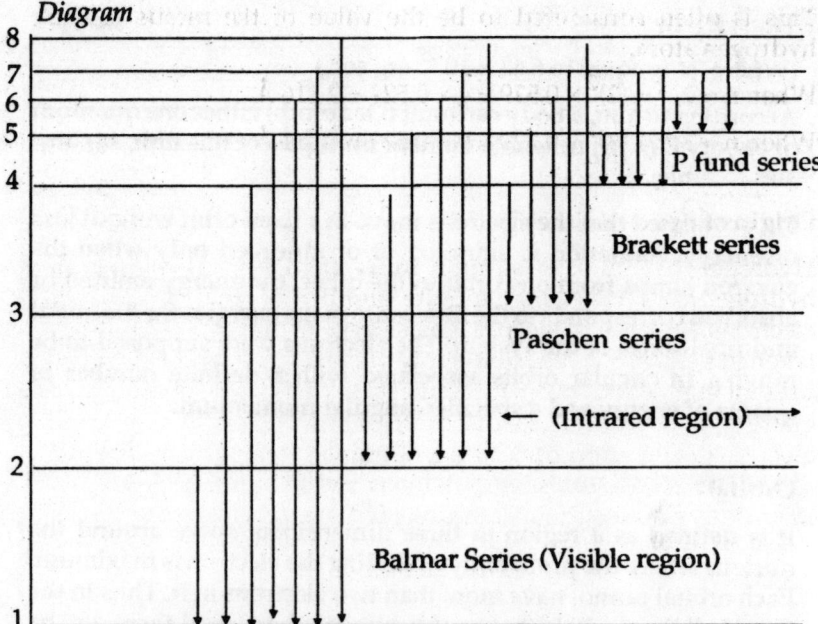

Fig. 4.4
Series of lines of hydrogen spectrum

Bohr's atomic model provides a satisfactory explanation for the various spectral lines formed in the hydrogen spectrum.

Quantum theory

According to quantum theory put forward by Planck a German physicist in 1900 and extended by Einstein 1905 energy is not lost or gained gradually but in units of hγ (known as quantum) where 'h' is a plank's constant and 'γ' is the frequency of the radiant energy.

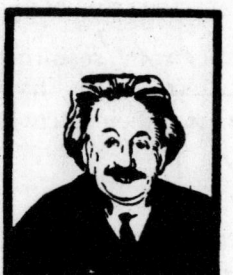

Elbert Einstein

The well-known author of the Theory of Relativity and the father of the equation $E = Mc^2$, which ultimately led to the discovery of the hydrogen bomb and the unlimited use of atomic energy for military, civil and industrial purposes. The matter-to-energy transformation gives 6,00,000 mile-tons of energy for 1 gram of matter transformed.

Thus, $E = h\gamma$

(Where 'h' is equal to 6.62×10^{-27} erg sec.)

According to him, a body can omit (Or absorb) either one quantum of energy E (= $h\gamma$) or whole number multiples of this unit, say $2h\gamma$, $3h\gamma$, ... $nh\gamma$.

He postulated that the electrons move in a fixed orbit without loss of energy. Radiation is emmited or or absorbed only when the electron jumps from one orbit to the other, the energy emitted or absorbed corresponds to the difference in the energies for the initial and final states of the system. The electrons were supposed to be moving in circular orbits associated with a definite number of quanta of energy and a specified angular momentum.

Orbital

It is defined as a region in three dimensional space around the nucleus where the probability of finding the electron is maximum. Each orbital cannot have more than two electrons in it. Thus in the first shell there will be only one orbital, in the second there will be four orbitals. Since the number of electrons in the first shell is two and in second eight respectively. Similarly, the third shell which has eighteen electrons will have nine orbitals and so on.

There are four types of orbitals e.g. s, p, d and f orbitals. 'S" orbital is spherical in shape with its centre at the nucleus of the atom. 'p' orbital, on the other hand, are dumb-bell shaped, the halves separated by a nodal plane where the probability of finding the electron is almost zero. The other types are 'd' and 'f' orbitals but these do not have any well defined shape.

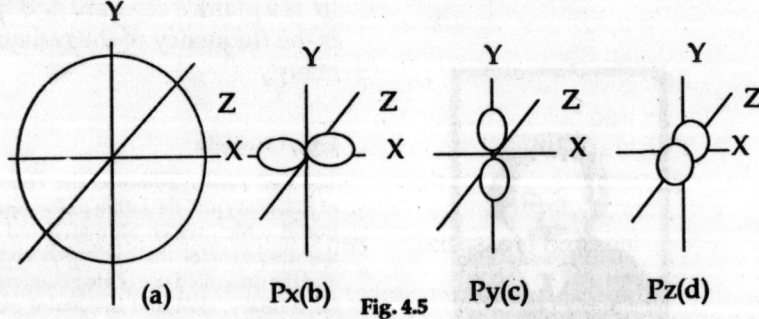

(a)   Px(b)   Fig. 4.5   Py(c)   Pz(d)

For conveninence and simplicity, the 1S and 2p orbitals are shown as in (a), (b), (c), (d).

Difference between an Orbit and Orbital

ORBIT	ORBITAL
1. It is well defined circular path around the nucleus in which the electron revolves. 2. It is circular in shape.	1. An orbital is the region of space around the nucleus where the probability of finding the electrons is maximum. s, p and d orbitals are spherical, dumb bell and double dumb-bell in shape respectively.
3. It represents that the electron moves around the nucleus in one plane.	It represents the three dimensional motion of electron round the nucleus.
4. It represents that the position as well as momentum of an electron can be known simultaneously with certainty. It is against Heisenberg's Uncertainty principle.	It represent that the position as well as the momentum of an electron cannot be known simultaneously with certainty. It is in accordance with Heisenberg's Uncertainty Principle.
5. The maximum number of electron in an orbit is $2n^2$ where 'n' is the number of the orbit.	The maximum number of electrons in an orbital is two.

Orbitals and Quantum Numbers

Quantum number gives the history of an electron in an atom. There is set of four quantum numbers: (i) Principal quantum number, (ii) Azimuthal quantum number, (iii) Magnetic quantum number and (iv) Spin quantum number.

(i) *Principal quantum number:* It is designated by 'n'. It gives an idea of the size. Its values are n = 1, 2, 3, ... (only positive integers). Large 'n' means large size. When n = 1, the electron belongs to K-shell and it belongs to L-shell when n = 2, and so on. It may be noted that the maimum number of electrons that can be present in a principal quantum number is $2n^2$. Lower value of 'n' represents that electron is near nucleus and is associated with small amount of energy.

(ii) Azimuthal quantum number or angular momentum quantum number. It gives the shape of an orbital and is designated as 'l'. It determines the energy associated with angular mometum of the electron moving around the nucleus. Its Values are $l = 0, 1, 2, 3$ ------- (n-1) (Zero and positive integers upto n-1)

(a) When n = 1, *l* has only one value i.e., 0. This means that the first shell (K-shell) is not divided further.

(b) When n = 2, *l* has two values i.e., 0 and 1. It means that second shell (L-shell) is composed of two sub-shells.

(c) When n = 3, *l* has three values, i.e. 0, 1 and (two) 2. It means there are three sub-shells in the third quantum number. The values of '*l*' (i.e., 0, 1, 2, 3) are designated by the letter s, p, d and f sub-shells respectively.

We designate different orbitals as follows:

n = 1, *l* = 0, 1s orbital (Where perfix '1' is the value of n)

n = 2, *l* = 0, 2s orbital (Where perfix '2' is the value of n)

n = 2, *l* = 1, 2p orbital (Where perfix '2' is the value of n)

(iii) **Magnetic quantum number.** It is designated by m. It gives the direction of the orbital in relation to the magnetic field in which it is placed. Its value depend upon the angular momentum quantum number '*l*'. For a given value of *l*, the possible values of m range from -*l* through zero to +*l* with a total value of (2*l* + *l*). Thus for *l* = 0, m can have only one value which is 0, for *l* = 1, m = -1, 0, + 1, for *l* = 2, m = -2, -1, 0, + 1, + 2 for *l* = 3, m = -3, -2, -1, 0, + 1, + 2, + 3. This shows that the number of orbitals which s, p, d and f sub-shell can have is 1,3,5 and 7, respectively.

(iv) *Spin quantum number:*

It is designated by S. It refers to the rotation of the electron about its axis in two opposite directions. Such a rotation is known as spin. It can have two values i.e., $+\frac{1}{2}$ and $-\frac{1}{2}$. As a rule when two electrons are present in an orbital, they have opposite spins (↑ ↓). This is called paring of spin.

Pauli exclusion principle

Austrian scientist, Wolfgang Pauli (1925) gave a rule which states that no two electrons in an atom can have the same set of four quantum numbers. It follows that any two electrons of an atom must differ in at least one quantum number. Because of Pauli's exclusion principle an orbital can contain only two electrons. It being understood that two electrons are spin paired. As a consequence of this principle, two is the maximum number of electrons permitted in one S-orbital, six in three p- orbitals and ten in the five d-orbitals. This can be seen in the Fig. 4.6.

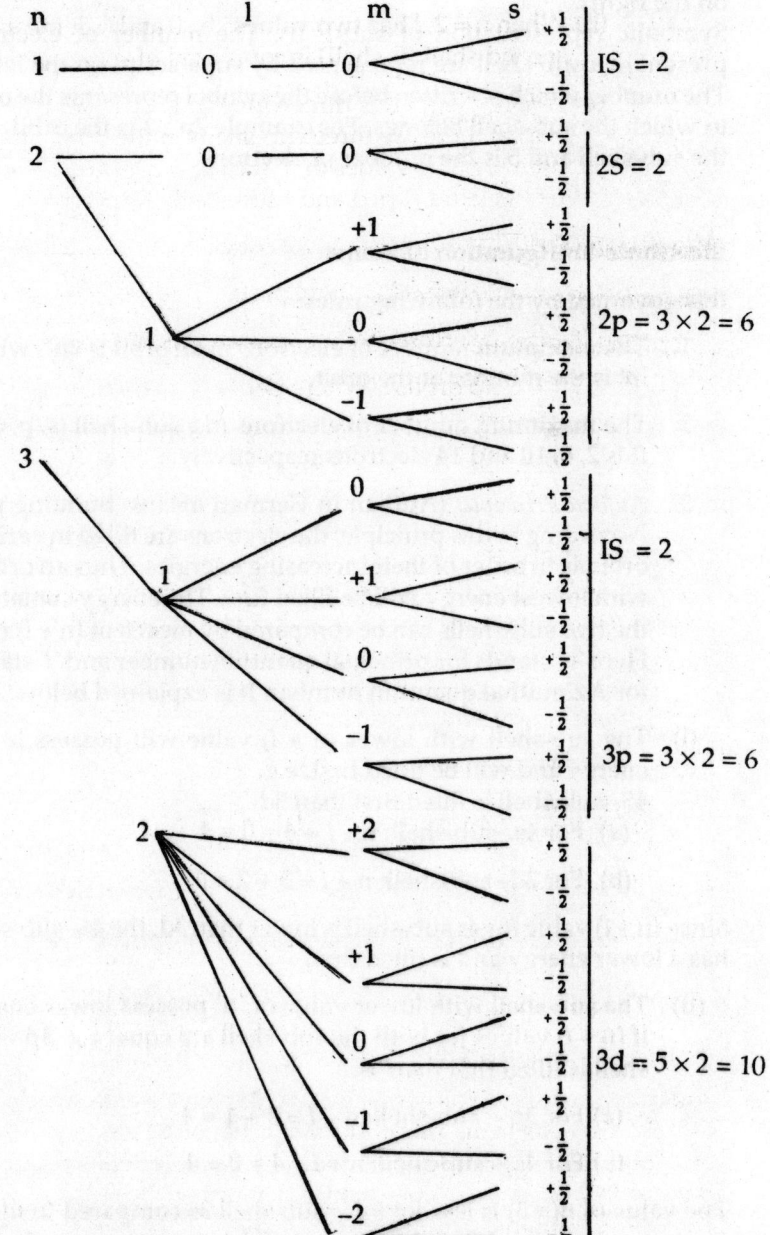

Fig. 4.6

Electrons in atom and quantum numbers. (The maximum number of electrons in which s, p, d subshell can accommodate is also shown on the right).

Symbolic representation of subshells. The number of electrons present in a sub-shell are represented by superscript on the letter. The number which is written before the symbol represents the orbit to which the sub-shell belongs. For example $2p^5$, 2 is the orbit, p is the sub-shell and 5 is the number of electrons.

Electronic configuration of atoms

It is governed by the following rules:

1. The maximum number of electrons in an orbit is $2n^2$, where 'n' is the number of the orbit.

2. The maximum number of electrons in a sub-shell (s, p, d or f) is 2, 6, 10 and 14 electrons respectively.

3. *Aufbau Principle:* (Aufbau in German means 'building up') According to this principle, the electrons are filled in various orbitals in order of their increasing energies. Thus an orbital with lowest energy will be filled first. The energy content of the two sub-shells can be compared by means of $(n + l)$ rule. Here 'n' stands for principal quantum number and 'l' stands for Azimuthal quantum number. It is explained below:

(i) The sub-shell with lower $(n + l)$ value will possess lower energy and will be filled first. e.g.
4S--sub-shell is filled first than 3d.
  (a) For 4s--sub-shell: $n + l = 4 + 0 = 4$

  (b) For 3d--sub-shell: $n + l = 3 + 2 = 5$.

Since $(n + l)$ value for 4s sub-shell is lower than 3d, the 4s--sub-shell has a lower energy and is filled first.

(ii) The sub-shell with lower value of 'n' possess lower energy if $(n + l)$ values for both the sub-shell are equal e.g. 3p--sub-shell is filled first than 4s.

  (a) For 3p -- sub-shell: $n + l = 3 + 1 = 4$

  (b) For 4s -- sub-shell: $n + l = 4 + 0 = 4$

The value of n($= 3$) is less for 3p -- sub-shell as compared to n($= 4$) for 4s -- sub-shell. Hence, 3p -- sub-shell has lower energy than 4s -- sub-shell and is filled first.

The energy of the various sub-shells increase in the following order.

$1S < 2S < 2p < 3S < 3p < 4S < 3d < 4p < 5s < 4d$-----------------

This order is diagrammatically illustrated below:

```
←——————  1S ←———
←——————  2S ←———
←——————  3S ←———  2p ←———
←——————  4S ←———  3p ←———
←——————  5S ←———  4p ←——— 3d ←———
←——————  6S ←———  5p ←——— 4d ←———
←——————  7S ←———  6p ←——— 5d ←——— 4f ←———
←——————  8S ←———  7p ←——— 6d ←——— 5f ←———
←——————  9S ←———  8p ←——— 7d ←——— 6f ←———
```

Order of filling up orbitals

(iii) **Hund's Rule of maximum multiplicity:**

According to this rule: No electron pairing takes place in p, d and f orbitals until each orbital in the given sub-shell contains one electron. As per Hund's rule, the electronic configuration of a few elements are given below:

Element	Atomic Number	Electronic configuration

		1s	2s	2p
N	7	↑↓	↑↓	↑ ↑ ↑
O	8	↑↓	↑↓	↑↓ ↑ ↑
F	9	↑↓	↑↓	↑↓ ↑↓ ↑

(iv) Fully filled orbitals and half-filled orbitals have extra stability (i.e. lower energy). Thus, the p^3, p^6, d^5, d^{10}, f^7 and f^{14} configuration which are either filled or half-filled, are more stable. Chromium and copper, therefore adopt the d^5

and d^{10} configurations in preference to the d^4 and d^9 configuration.

Element	Atomic Number	Electronic Configuration
Cr	24	$1S^2, 2S^2 p^6, 3S^2 p^6 d^5, 4S^1$
Cu	29	$1S^2, 2S^2 p^6, 3S^2 p^6 d^{10}, 4S^1$

Electronic configuration of elements with atomic number 1 to 20:

Element	Atomic Number	Electronic configuration
H	1	$1S^1$
He	2	$1S^2$
Li	3	He $2S^1$
Be	4	$-2S^2$
B	5	$-2S^2.2p^1$
C	6	$-2S^2.2p^2$
N	7	$-2S^2.2p^3$
O	8	$-2S^2.2p^4$
F	9	$-2S^2.2p^5$
Ne	10	$-2S^2.2p^6$
Na	11	$-Ne\ 3S^1$
Mg	12	$-3S^2$
Al	13	$-3S^2.3p^1$
Si	14	$-3S^2.3p^2$
P	15	$-3S^2.3p^3$
S	16	$-3S^2.3p^4$
Cl	17	$-3S^2.3p^5$
Ar	18	$-3S^2.3p^6$
K	19	Ar $4S^1$
Ca	20	$-4S^2$

QUESTIONS

1. (a) State the essential features of Bohr's model of the atom.
   (S 1989)

   (b) Name the four quantum numbers. What does each quantum number describe? (S 1989)

2. (a) Describe briefly the structure of the atom.
   (b) The nucleus of the atom of an element consists of 12 neutrons and 12 electrons, Find

   (i) Atomic Weight
   (ii) Atomic Number
   (iii) Electro valency of element. (W 1988)

3. (a) Describe briefly the structure of atom. Explain clearly the various terms involved.
   (b) Write the electronic configuration and also give the valency of the atom with the following atomic number:
   (i) 12   (ii) 17   (iii) 19   (W 1989)

4. Explain in briefly the origin of spectral lines.

5. Name various series of lines which make up the hydrogen spectrum. Draw the necessary diagram.

OBJECTIVE TYPE QUESTIONS

6. Select the correct answer:

   (a) The maximum number of electrons which can occupy p-subshells.
   (i) 2,   (ii) 3,   (iii) 4,   (iv) 5,   (v) 6

   (b) The model of an atom consisting of a dense positively charge nucleus surrounded by electrons is due to (i) N. Bohr (ii) Rutherford (iii) J.J. Thomson (iv) M. Plank.

   (c) Which one of the following orbital is spherically symmetrical?
   (i) 3S (ii) 3p (iii) 3d (iv) 4f.

   (d) In the ground state, the electron is
   (i) Nearest to the nucleus (ii) Farthest from the nucleus (iii) In the second shell.

   (e) The maximum electron capacity of any orbital is (i) 2 (ii) 8 (iii) 18 (iv) 32

ANSWERS

6. (a) v   (b) i   (c) i   (d) i   (e) i.

Chapter V

Periodicity of Elements

Mendeleev a great Russian Chemist stated in 1869 his periodic law. Proporties of the elements are periodic function of their atomic weights i.e., if elements are arranged in order of their atomic weights, similar elements are repeated at regular intervals or periods. Mendeleev arranged the element then known, in the order of increasing atomic weights in the form of a table called Mendeleev's Periodic Table chart 5.1.

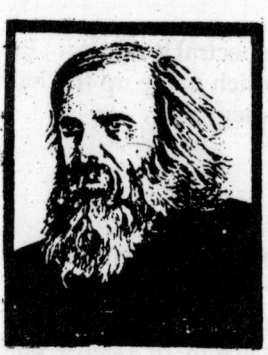

There were certain defects in this table and is therefore not discussed here.

Dimitri Ivanovitch Mendeleev

(1834-1907)

A Russian Chemist who was Professor of Chemistry in the University of St. Petersberg. He is famous for his Periodic Law and the development of Petroleum and other industries in Russia.

It has been replaced by long form of the Periodic Table.

Periodicity of elements: Long form of the periodic Table and classification of elements on the basis of electronic configuration.

Modern Periodic law: It states that when the elements are arranged in order of their increasing atomic number, similar elements are repeated after regular intervals. The modern periodic table is based on this law. The most popular versions of the modern periodic table is the long-form-Chart 5.2. This table has the following features:

1. In this table there are eighteen vertical columns consisting of sixteen groups. The sixteen groups are designated as IA, IIA, . . . VIIA: IB, IIB, . . . VIIB; VIII and zero.
2. Elements of sub-group IA, IIA . . . . VIIA have only outer shell incomplete. Each one of their inner shells is complete. These are called normal elements.

3. The elements of sub-group IB, IIB, ...VIIB and VIII have their outermost, as well as penultimate shell incomplete. These are called transitional elements.

4. Elements of sub-group zero have all their shells complete. These do not show any reactivity and are termed as normal gases.

5. Horizontal rows are called periods. There are seven periods in the table:

   (i) The first period is of two elements (H ------ He)
   (ii) Second and third are two short periods of eight elements each. (Li ---- Ne) and (Na ---- Ar)
   (iii) Fourth and fifth are long periods of eighteen elements each, while sixth is a long period of thirty two elements.
   (iv) Seventh is an incomplete period and contains nineteen elements which are radioactive.

6. Noblel gases are grouped at the extreme right of the periodic table.

7. Lanthanide and actinide have been grouped separately and placed at the bottom. In the sixth period, elements with atomic number 58 to 71 resemble in properties with Lanthanum and have been grouped with Lanthanum (At. No. 57) and are called Lanthanides. Similarly in the seven period, elements with atomic number (90 - 103) resemble in properties with Actinium (At. No. 89) and are called Actinides.

8. As we move across the period from left to right the metallic character become less and less while non-metallic character increases progressively.

9. In the table, the elements of the same period show a regular gradation in properties both physical and chemical eg. in 2nd period.

   (i) We start with a electropositive element and we end with a electronegative element.

   (ii) The basic character of the oxide decreases and the acid character of the oxide increases. eg.

Na_2O, MgO	Al_2O_3
Basic *oxide* of decreasing intensity	Amphoteric oxide

CHART 5.1

MENDELEEV'S PERIODIC TABLE

Group	I A	I B	II A	II B	III A	III B	IV A	IV B	V A	V B	VI A	VI B	VII A	VII B	VIII	0
Period 1	H I 1.008												H 1 1.008			He 2 4.003
" 2	Li 3 0.940		Be 4 9.09			B 5 10.82		C 6 12.01		N 7 14.01		O 8 16.00		F 9 19.00		Ne 10 10.123
" 3	Na 11 23.00		Mg 12 24.32			Al 13 26.07		Si 14 28.06		P 15 31.02		S 16 32.06		Cl 17 35.46		A 18 39.944
" 4 First Series	K 19 39.10		Ca 20 40.48		Sc 21 45.10		Ti 22 47.90		V 23 50.95		Cr 24 52.01		Mn 25 54.93		Fe 26 55.84 Co 27 55.94 Ni 28 58.69	
Second Series		CU 29 63.57		Zn 30 65.38		Ga 31 65.72		Ge 32 72.69		As 33 74.91		Se 34 78.96		Br 35 79.92		Kr 36 83.7
" 5 First Series	Rb 37 85.48		Sr 38 87.63		Y 39 88.92		Zr 40 91.22		Nb 41 92.91		Mo 42 95.95		Tc 43 97.8		Ru 44 101.7 Rb 45 102.91 Pd 46 106.7	
Second Series		Ag 47 107.88		Cd 48 112.4		In 49 114.76		Sn 50 118.70		Sb 51 121.76		Te 52 127.61		I 53 126.92		Xe 54 131.3

Periods 6 and 7

6	First Series	Cs 55 132.91	Ba 56 137.36	La 57* 138.92	Hf 72 178.6	Ta 73 180.88	W 74 183.92	Re 75 186.31	Os 76 190.2	Ir 77 193.1	Pt 78 195.23
	Second Series	Au 79 197.2	Hg 80 200.62	Tl 81 204.39	Pb 82 207.21	Bi 83 209.00	Po 84 210	At 85 —	Rn 86 222		
7	Fr 87	Ra 88 266.05	Ac 89** 229	Th 90 232.12	Pa 91 231	U 92 238.07					

*Rare Earth (Lanthanides) 58 · 71

Ce 58 140.13	Pr 59 140.9	Nd 60 144.27	Pm 61 147	Sm 62 150.4	Eu 63 152	Gd 64 156.9
Tb 65 159.2	Dy 66 162.47	Ho 67 163.5	Er 68 167.2	Tm 69 169.4	Yb 70 173.04	Lu 71 174.90

**ACTINIDES

Th 90 232.12	Pa 91 231	U 92 238.07	Np 93 231	Pu 94 242	Am 95 243	Cm 96 243	Bk 97 245	Cf 98 246
Es 99	Fm 100	Md 101	No 102	Lw 103				

CHART 5.2.

LONG FORM PERIODIC TABLE

Representative Elements ——————————— Representative Elements

Periods \ Groups	1A	IIA	IIIB	IVB	VB	VIB	VIIB	VIII	VIII	VIII	IB	IIB	IIIA	IVA	VA	VIA	VIIA	0
1	H 1																	He 2
2	Li 3	Be 4											B 5	C 6	N 7	O 8	F 9	Ne 10
3	Na 11	Mg 12											Al 13	Si 14	P 15	S 16	Cl 17	Ar 18
4	K 19	Ca 20	Sc 21	Ti 22	V 23	Cr 24	Mn 25	Fe 26	Co 27	Ni 28	Cu 29	Zn 30	Ga 31	Ge 32	As 33	Se 34	Br 35	Kr 36
5	Rb 37	Sr 38	Y 39	Zr 40	Nb 41	Mo 42	Tc 43	Ru 44	Rh 45	Pd 46	Ag 47	Cd 48	In 49	Sn 50	Sb 51	Te 52	I 53	Xe 54
6	Cs 55	Ba 56	La 57	Hf 72	Ta 73	W 74	Re 75	Os 76	Ir 77	Pt 78	Au 79	Hg 80	Tl 81	Pb 82	Bi 83	Po 84	At 85	Rn 86
7	Fr 87	Ra 88	Ac 89	Ku 104	Ha 105													

Transition Elements

Lanthanide Series —	Ce 58	Pr 59	Nd 60	Pm 61	Sm 62	Eu 63	Gd 64	Tb 65	Dy 66	Ho 67	Er 68	Tm 69	Yb 70	Lr 71
Actinide Series —	Th 90	Pa 91	U 92	Np 93	Pu 94	Am 95	Cm 96	Bk 97	Cf 98	Es 99	Fm 100	Md 101	No 102	Lw 103

Long form of the periodic table. (The heavy line approximately separates the metallic elements, to the left, from non-metallic elements, to the right. Representative elements 'to the left' come under s-block, representative elements, except He 'to the right' come under p-block, transition elements come under d-block, and lanthanides and actinides come under f-block).

$$\frac{\text{SiO}_2,\ \text{P}_2\,\text{O}_5,\ \text{SO}_3,\ \text{Cl}_2\,\text{O}_7}{\text{Acidic oxide of increasing intensity}}$$

10. The elements placed in the same group show certain regularities.

11. In the table element show gradation of valency.

12. *Diagonal Relationship:* On moving diagonally across the periodic table the elements show certain similarities. These are usually weaker than the similarities within a group but are quite pronounced in the case of few elements given below:

IA	IIA	IIIA	IVA
Li	Be	B	C
Na	Mg	Al	Si

Classification of elements on the basis of electronic configurations

From the electronic configuration of these elements we find that all elements having the same number of electrons in the valence shell have similar properties. Hence, cause of periodicity is the recurrence of similar electronic configurations. The properties of the elements get repeated after intervals of 2, 8, 8, 18, 18, and 32 because similar electronic configurations occur only after these intervals.

On the basis of electronic configuration the elements have been classified into four blocks in the long-form of the periodic table. These blocks of elements are: (i) S-block, (ii) p-block, (iii) d-block, (iv) f-block.

(i) *S-block Elements:* These elements belong to group IA (alkali metals such as Li, Na and K) and group IIA (alkaline earth metals such as Be, Mg, Ca and Sr) and have outermost electronic configuration as ns^1 and ns^2 respectively.

Elements of s-block have completely filled inner orbitals.

Example: Na -- $1S^2, 2S^2.\ 2P^6, 3S^1$
$\qquad\qquad$ Mg -- $iS^2, 2S^2.\ 2P^6, 3S^2$.

(ii) *p-block Elements:* The elements of group IIIA to VIIA and zero group with the outermost electronic configuration varying between $ns^2\ np^1$ and $ns^2\ np^6$ are called p-block elements. Elements present in zero group with $ns^2\ np^6$ electronic configuration come at the end of this block. These elements are called noble gases. Elements of p-block have completely filled inner orbitals.

Examples: $B - 1S^2, 2S^2. 2P^1$
                 $F - 1S^2, 2S^2. 2P^5.$

(iii)   *d-block Elements (Transition elements):* Elements with atoms in which two outermost shells are incomplete. The elements present in the group IIIB to IIB and VIII in the centre of the periodic table with common electronic configuration $(n - 1)$ d^{1-10} ns^{0-2} are known as elements of d-block elements. In case of these elements, n is 4, 5, or 6 and electrons are being filled in 3d, 4d, or 5d orbitals. They make up three complete rows of 10 elements and an incomplete fourth row in the periodic table. The d-block elements have characteristics which are intermediate between those of the s and p-block elements, and hence are called transition elements.

Examples. $Cr - 1S^2, 2S^2. 2P^6, 3S^2. 3P^6. 3d^5, 4S^1$
                 $Cu - 1s^2, 2S^2. 2P^6, 3S^2. 3P^6. 3d^{10}, 4S^1$

(iv)   *f-block Elements (inner transition elements):* Elements having three outermost shells incomplete. These elements are arranged in the two rows at the bottom of the periodic table. The first row includes rare earth of lanthanide elements from atomic number 58 to 71. The second row includes actinide elements from atomic number 90 to 103. Lanthanides and actinides have incomplete 4f or 5f orbitals respectively. In addition they also have incomplete (n-1)d orbitals. The f-block elements also refered to as inner transition elements because in case of these elements, their antipenultimate (third from outermost) shell is being expan- ded from 18 to 32 by the addition of f-electrons.

Examples: $Ce - 1S^2, 2S^2 2P^6, 3S^2 3P^6 3d^{10}, 4S^2 4p^6 4d^{10}, 5S^2 5p^6,$
                 $4f^2, 6S^2$

                 $Ac - 1S^2, 2S^2 2P^6, 3S^2 3p^6 3d^{10}, 4S^2 4p^6 4d^{10}, 5S^2 5p^6,$
                 $4f^{14} 5d^{10}, 6S^2 6p^6 6d^1, 7S^2$

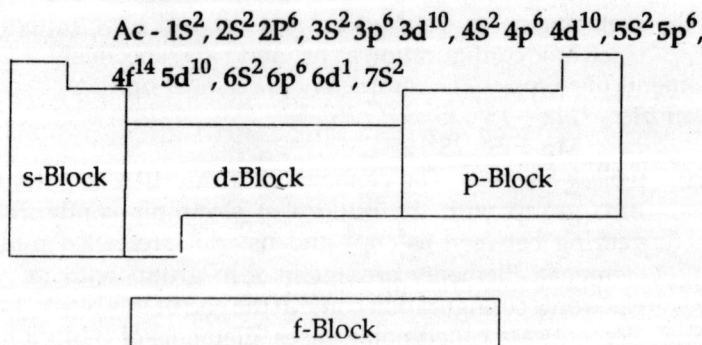

Fig. 5.2   Division of periodic table into four blocks.

Fig. 5.2 Shows that the elements in which the s, p, d & f orbitals are being filled up are grouped naturally in the long form of the periodic table.

Advantages of the long form of the periodic table

1. Elements have been arranged in the increasing order of their atomic number which is more fundamental property than atomic weight.

2. It relates the position of an element in the table to its electronic configuration more clearly.

3. It reflects the similarities, differences and trends in chemical properties more clearly.

4. It is an easy chart to remember and reproduce.

5. Active metals, non metals, metalloids, transition elements, lanthanide and actinide are clearly seperated in the periodic table.

6. There is a logical seperation of sub-group in it. The element found in any of its vertical column resemble closely with each other.

7. The position of isotopes is justified.

8. The position of misfits in the Mendeleev periodic table when atomic weight is the basis of classification is explained on the basis of rising atomic number. For example placing of Ar (At. No. -- 18) before K (At. No. --- 19) extra, can be easily justified.

TRENDS OF PROPERTIES

1. *Valency:* In s and p-block elements in each short period valency with respect to oxygen increases from 1 in group IA to 7 in group VIIA, but in respect of hydrogen and chlorine the valency first increases from 1 in group IA to 4 in group VI A and then decreases to 1 in group VIIA.

   For example in elements of third short period going from left to right.

   Oxides are: Na_2O MgO Al_2O_3 SlO_2 P_2O_5 SO_3 Cl_2O_7

   Valency is: 1   2   3   4   5   6   7

Therefore the valency of the elements with respect to oxygen corresponds to the group number.

Hydrides are: NaH MgH₂ AlH₃ SiH₄ PH₃ H₂S HCl

Valency is :   1   2   3   4   3   2   1

In the same group all the elements have same valency.

Variable Valency

d-block elements: In addition to using the electrons in the outermost energy levels for compound formation, d-block elements can also use a variable number of inner d electrons for this purpose, as such show variable valency but all of them have a common Valency of 2.

Example: Element Valency
          Fe   3, 2 in the formation of ferric
                   and ferrous compounds.
          Cu   2, 1 in the formation of curpric
                   and cuprous compounds.

f-block elements: They also exhibt variable valencies.

Noble gases: They are zero valent.

2. *Oxidation number:* It is defined as the charge which an atom of the element appears to have in a given molecule when electrons are counted according to certain orbitrary rules. The following rules and conventions are used in denoting oxidation numbers to the various elements.

   (a) The oxidation number of all elements in the uncombined state is zero.

   (b) The oxidation number of an ion is the same as its charge. The oxidation number of L^+, Ca^{2+} and Al^{3+} ions are +1, +2, and +3 while those of Cl^-, SO_4^{2-}, and PO_4^{3-} ions are -1, -2, and -3 respectively.

   (c) The sum of the oxidation numbers of all the atoms in the formula of the neutral compound is zero.

   (d) In all hydrogen compounds (except hydrides of active metals such as Li, Na and Ca) the oxidation number of hydrogen per atom is +1.

   (e) In all oxygen compounds (except hydrogen peroxide and other peroxides) the oxidation number of oxygen is to taken to be -2.

With the above rules and conventions, it is possible to find out oxidation number (state) of any element in a compound, provided the oxidation number (state) of other elements are known.

Calculation of oxidation number of chromium in potassium dichromate. We know oxidation number of potassium is +1 and that of oxygen is -2 per atom. Let the oxidation number of chromium be x.

$$K_2Cr_2O_7$$

Sum of oxidation number = 0 i.e. +2 +2x - 14 = 0, x = 6 Therefore oxidation number of chromium in potassium dichromate is 6.

Calculation of oxidation number of sulphur in sodium sulphate. The oxidation number of sodium is +1 and that of oxygen is -2 per atom. Let oxidation number of sulphur be x. By rule (c) the sum of oxidation numbers of all the atoms in the formula of a neutral compound is zero.

The sum of the oxidation numbers = 0

$$Na_2S\ O_4$$

$$2 + x - 8 = 0$$

$$\therefore x = 6$$

Thus the oxidation number of sulphur in sodium sulphate is 6.

As a rule to which there are few exception the highest positive oxidation number of an element is the same as its group number while the highest negative oxidation number = 8-group number. Thus, the highest negative oxidation number of nitrogen is $8 - 5 = 3$ which it displays in ammonia. The other oxidation number of nitrogen in its oxides will be +1 in N_2O; +2 in NO; +4 in NO_2 and +5 in N_2O_5.

Oxidation number concept and the Periodic Table

   (a)   *S-block elements:*

       (i) Elements of group I A show a maximum oxidation number of +1, whereas elements of group II A show maximum oxidation number of +2.

   (b)   *p-block elements:*

Elements of p-block exhibt more than one oxidation number e.g.

       (i) Elements of group III A such as Indium show an oxidation number of +1 and +3.

(ii) Elements of group IV A exhibt an oxidation number of +2 and +4.

(iii) Elements of V A group show an oxidation number of +3, +5 and -3.

(iv) Elements of VI A group show oxidation number of +2, +4, +6 and -2 while

(v) Some elements of VII A group show an oxidation number of +1, +3, +5, +7, and -1.

(c) d-block elements exhibit a large number of oxidation number e.g.

Element	Sc	Ti	V
Outer electronic configuration	$3d^1 4S^2$	$3d^2 4S^2$	$3d^3 4S^2$
Stable oxidation number	+3	+3, +4	+3, +4, +5

(d) f-block elements also exhibit multiple oxidation number e.g., uranium shows +3, +4, +5, +6.

3. *Atomic size:* It is difficult to determine the exact size of an atom. However, one can estimate the approximate radii of atoms by knowing the distance between the atoms in molecule. In general, atomic radius decreases while going from left to right across the periodic table and increases while going from top to bottom. This is shown in table below:

Atomic radii of elements in second period.

Atomic number	3	4	5	6	7	8	9
Element	Li	Be	B	C	N	O	F
Atomic radius Å	1.23	0.89	0.80	0.77	0.74	0.74	0.72

Atomic radii of alkali metals

Atomic number	Element	Atomic radius (Å)
3	Li	1.23
11	Na	1.57
19	K	2.03
37	Rb	2.16
55	Cs	2.35

Explanations: The decrease in atomic radius across a period arises from the effect of increasing nuclear charge while electrons are being added to the same shell. As the nuclear charge increases, electrons are attracted to a greater extent and atomic size decreases. The increase in the atomic radius in going down a group is due to the presence of increasing number of electron shells. Although the nuclear charge increases as we go down a group, its effect will be little compared to the dominating effect of a new shell of electrons being added.

QUESTIONS

1. The chemical properties of the elements are a periodic function of their atomic numbers. Illustrate this statement by reference to the first few elements. Show how electronic structure account for the periodicity of the properties.

2. What do you understand by s, p, d and f-blocks of element?

3. Which are the transition elements in the periodic table and how are they characterised in terms of electronic configuration?

4. Describe the structural features of the long form of periodic table.

5. Discuss the variations in atomic sizes amongst the elements of (i) group and (ii) periods of the periodic table.

6. Name the four blocks of elements in the periodic table and indicate the main difference in their electronic structure. Give one example of each type of element.

7. What are the trends in valency in the periodic table?

8. In the period of elements in the periodic table, atomic radii ordinarily decreases with increasing atomic number. Why is it so?

9. Mention the advantages of the long form of the periodic table.

10. What is the trend of the following properties in the periodic table (a) valency, (b) atomic size and (c) oxidation number.

11. Write note on s, p, d and f-block elements. (W-1989)

12.   a. What is the electrovalency concept of Valency. Explain with eamples electrovalency and Co-ordinate valency.

    b. The nucleus of the atom of an element consists of 12 neutrons and 12 electrons find:

    a) Atomic Weight b)Atomic number and c) Electrovalency of element. (S-1990)

    c. Select the correct words:

    (i) Charge on a proton is equal to charge on electron/neutron.

    (ii) Isotopes have same atomic number/atomic weight.

    (iii) Isobars have different atomic number/atomic weight.

    (iv) Electrons are stationary/moving.round the nucleus.

    (v) Sodium chloride is an electrovalent/covalent compound. (S-1988)

OBJECTIVE-TYPE QUESTIONS

13. *Fill in the blanks*

    (i) d-block elements are placed in between--------and------.

    (ii) Electron effinities of---------group element is zero.

    (iii) Sodium ion has----------radius than chlorine ion.

    (iv) The number of elements present in first period of periodic table is------------.

    (v) Li, Na and K are present in ------- group of the periodic table.

14. **Tick mark the correct answers.**

(i) Long form of periodic table is based on the properties of elements as a function of

a) atomic weight   b) atomic number   c) atomic volume.

(ii) On decending a vertical group (periodic table) the size of the atom

a) Increases   b) decreases   c) does not change.

(iii) The number of elements in the sixth period of the periodic table is:

a) 8   b)   18   c) 32

ANSWERS

12. b. (a) 24 (b) 12 (c) 2

    c. i) electron ii) same atomic number iii) different atomic number iv) moving round the nucleus v) electrovalent.

13. i) s and p ii) zero iii) lower iv) 2 v) I A

14. i) b ii) a iii) c

Chapter VI

Osmosis and Osmotic Pressure

Semipermeable membrane

In the middle of the eighteenth century it was observed that there are certain memberanes which when placed between a solution and the solvent present in it allow passage across to the solvent molecules but do not permit solute molecules or ions to pass through. These memberanes are said to be semipermable. Examples of semipermeable membrane; parchment paper, cellophane, animal membranes (pig bladder). A more efficient membrane is a film of copper ferrocyanide. It is formed in the walls of a porous pot by allowing solution of copper sulphate and potassium ferrocyanide to meet inside the walls **Fig. 6.1.**

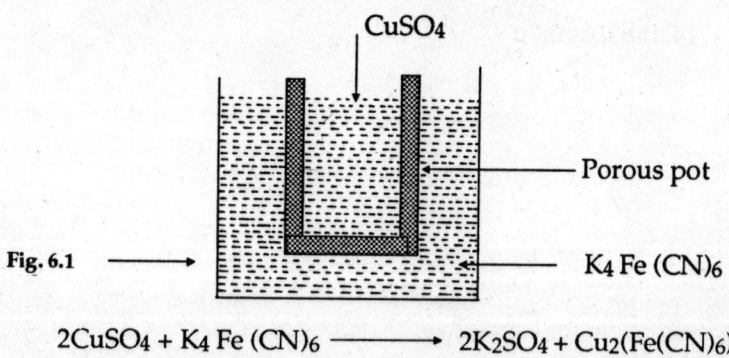

$CuSO_4$

Porous pot

Fig. 6.1

$K_4 Fe (CN)_6$

$$2CuSO_4 + K_4 Fe (CN)_6 \longrightarrow 2K_2SO_4 + Cu_2(Fe(CN)_6)$$

Phenomenon of Osmosis (Greek; Osmos = a push)

The phenomenon of the passage of pure solvent into a solution through a semipermeable memberane is called Osmosis. Osmosis can also take place between solutions of different concentration separated by a semipermeable membrane. In such cases, the solvent flows from the solutions of low solute concentration to that of higher concentration.

Demonstration of the phenomenon of osmosis and to prove the existence of osmotic pressure. Experiment due to Abbe Nollet (1748). We take a thistle funnel and tie round its neck a piece of pig bladder. Partly fill it with a 1% solution of cane sugar and make it stand vertically with the bladder wall immeresed in a breaker of water as shown in Fig. 6.2. The level of the solution inside the funnel tube will be found to slowly rise, owing to osmosis of pure water into the tube, until finally it becomes stationary at a certain height depending upon the concentration of the solution.

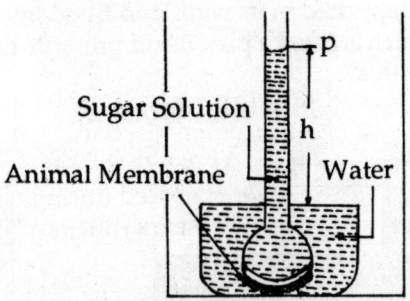

Fig. 6.2: Experiment to illustrate the existence of Osmotic Pressure.

In the experiment passage of the solvent into the solution continues, until the hydrostatic pressure of the column of the solution is just sufficient to stop the entry of more solvent into the solution. The solvent molecules exert a pressure on the solution which is counter-balanced by weight of the hydrostatic column h, of the solution. This pressure is known as the osmotic pressure of the system. Solution/Semipermeable membrane/Pure solvent.

Osmotic Pressure

The extra pressure to be applied on the solution side necessary to counter act the pressure due to osmosis when the solution and the solvent are seperated by a semipermeable membrane is a measure of the osmotic pressure of solution or it may be defined as the additional pressure which has to be applied on the solution to prevent the osmosis of the pure solvent into it.

Osmotic pressure is given by the relationship
$$\pi = \frac{n\beta . RT}{V}$$
Where π is the osmotic pressure

'$n\beta$' is the moles of solute in V liters of the solution.

'R' is the gas constant and

'T' is the absolute temperature.

Measurement of Osmotic pressure

Berkeley and Hartley's method for determining the Osmotic pressure of the dilute solution.

The apparatus (Fig. 6.3) used consists of a porous pot containing copper ferrocyanide deposited in its walls and fitted into a bronze or steel cylinder to which is fitted a piston and pressure gauze. The porous pot is fitted with a

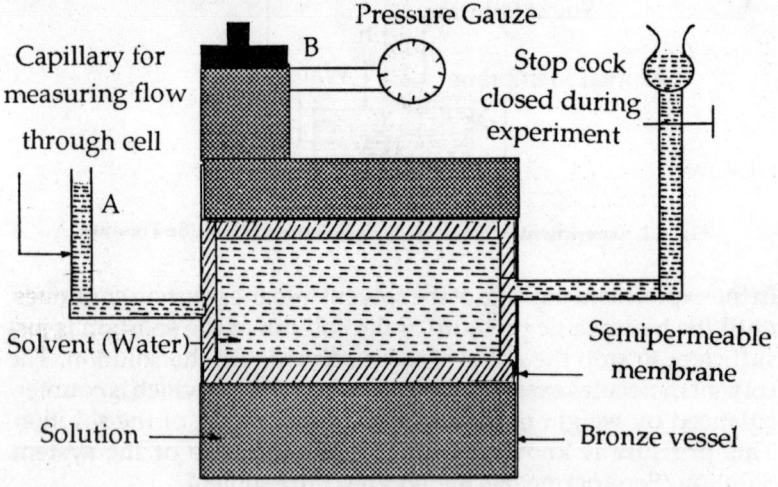

Pressure Gauze

Capillary for measuring flow through cell

Stop cock closed during experiment

A

Solvent (Water)

Semipermeable membrane

Solution

Bronze vessel

Fig. 6.3: Berkeley and Hartley method.

Osmotic pressure = pressure required at B to maintain water level incapillary tube at A

reservoir on the right and a capillary indicator on the left. Water is put in the porous pot while the bronze cylinder is filled with the solution of which the osmotic pressure is to be measured. Water placed in the porous pot tends to pass into the solution through the semipermeable membrane with the result that the capillary indicator moves downwards. External pressure is now applied by the piston so that the level in the capillary indicator remains stationary. This pressure which is equal to the osmotic pressure is read off on the pressure gauge.

Example: Calculate the osmotic pressure of solution containing 0.1 mole of solute per litre at 273k.

Osmotic pressure is given by the relationship

$$\pi = \frac{n\beta \times RT}{V}$$

Where 'π' is the osmotic pressure

'$n\beta$' is the mole of solute in V liters of the solution

'R' is the gas constant and

'T' is the absolute temperature, substituting the values

$$\pi = \frac{0.1 \times 0.082 \times 273}{1} = 2.22 \text{ atm.}$$

QUESTIONS

1. Explain the term Osmosis, Osmotic pressure and Semi-permeable membrane.

2. What is meant by term Osmotic pressure. Describe Berkeley and Hartley's method for the determination of Osmotic pressure of solution.

3. How can a semipermeable membrane be prepared and used for the determination of osmotic pressure of a solution of sucrose.

4. What is Osomotic pressure? How it is determined? (S - 1990)

5. Calculate the osmotic pressure at 25°c of a 5% solution of urea. Solution:

    We have in this case

    V = 0.1 litre

    w = 5 gm.

    M = 60

    R = 0.082 litre atmosphere per degree

    T = 298° absolute

Substituting these values in the equation

$$\pi = \frac{n\,\beta \times RT}{V}$$

$$= \frac{1}{0.1} \times \frac{5}{60} \times 0.082 \times 298 = 20.4 \text{ atmosphere.}$$

6. A solution of sucrose (molecular mass 342g/mole) is prepared by dissolving 68.4 g of it per litre of solution. What is its osmotic pressure at 300k, R = 0.082 litre atmosphere per degree per mole.

7. Calculate the osmotic pressure of 5% solution of glucose ($C_6H_{12}O_6$) at $18^\circ C$(R = 0.082 litre-atm./degree).

8. Calculate the osmotic pressure of 19% solution of cane sugar (M. Wt. 342) at $27^\circ C$. (R = 0.082 litre-atm./degree)

9. Calculate the osmotic pressure of 10% solution of cane sugar at $15^\circ C$ (C = 12, H = 1, O = 16 are the atomic weights) (S 1990)

10. Write note on phenomenon of Osmosis (W 1989)

OBJECTIVE TYPE QUESTIONS

11. *Fill in the blanks:*

    (i) A ----------allows only the solvent molecules and not the soluble particles to pass through it.

    (ii) The spontaneous flow of a solvent into a solution or from a solution of low cocentration to that of higher concentration through a semipermeable membrane is known as -------.

    (iii) -------- is defined as the equivalent of extra pressure which must be applied to a solution to prevent the flow of solvent into it through a semipermeable membrane.

ANSWERS

6. 4.92 atm.   7. 6.64 atm.   8. 13.6 atm.

9. 6.8 atm.

11. (i) Semipermeable membrane

    (ii) Osmosis

    (iii) Osmotic pressure.

Chapter VII

Colloids

The colloidal state of matter.

Thomas Graham in 1861 made a distinction between solutes which diffused rapidly through vegetable or animal membrane and those which diffused very slowly. First type of substance he named crystalloids e.g. sugar, salt, copper sulphate, urea etc., while he called the other group colloids (Greek Kolla = glue, idos = like) e.g. gum, silicic acid, starch, gelatin, egg albumen. Crystalloids in solution yield very small particles (ions or molecules) which can easily pass through the pores of a membrane where as a colloids give bigger particles which cannot diffuse through the membrane. This

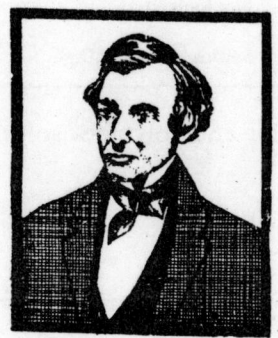

Thomas Graham (1805-1869)

A Scottish Chemist who is regarded as the "father of Colloidal Chemistry". He enunciated the Law of Gaseous diffusion and did remarkable work on diffusion of substances in solution.

implies that by varying the particle size by adopting suitable methods, a crystalloids may be made to behave like a colloid and vice versa. For example, Sodium salts of long chain fatty acids (the soap) show colloidal character in water in which they are very sparingly soluble but crystalloids character in alcohol in which they are freely soluble. The term 'colloidal substance' has therefore been discarded in favour of colloidal state into which almost every substance can be brought by suitable means. Distinction between a True solution and Colloidal solution is given in **Table 7.1**.

Table 7.1

	Property	True solution	Colloidal solution
1.	Nature	Homogeneous	Heterogeneous
2.	Size of particles	1×10^{-7} cm.	1×10^{-4} cm. to 1×10^{-7} cm.
3.	Filterability	Passes through ordinary filter paper, vegetable and animal membrane	Passes through ordinary filter paper but not through vegetable of animal membrane
4.	Diffusion	Diffuses readily	Diffuses slowly
5.	Tyndall effect	Does not show Tyndall effect	Shows Tyndall effect
6.	Electrical charge	Uncharged	Charged either positively or negatively
7.	Brownian movement	Does not show	Shows Brownian movement
8.	Ionisation	May be ionised	Not ionised
9.	Setting	Does not settle	Settles in a contrifuge

Distinction between a colloidal dispersion and Polymeric solution is given in Table 7.2.

Table 7.2

	Property	Colloidal dispersion	Polymeric solution
1.	Size	1×10^{-4} cm to 1×10^{-7} cm consists of atoms or small molecules. For example a gold sol. may contains particles of various sizes having several atoms. Sulphur sol. consists of particles containing a thousand or so of S_8-sulphur molecules.	Have large size and themselves large molecule contain large number of atoms. They are also called macro molecular colloids. These dispersions resemble true solution in may ways
2.	Molecular masses	Low	High, ranging from thousand to millions.

	Property	Colloidal dispersion	Polymeric solution
3.	Bonding forces	Particles are held together by Vander Waals forces.	The particles of colloidal dimensions are individual molecules which are held by true chemical bonds. Example of natural polymers are starch, cellulose and protein. Some man made polymers are polyethylene, synthetic rubber, polystyrene, nylon etc. etc.

Types of colloidal system

Finely divided particles or any substance with diameter lying between 1×10^{-7} to 1×10^{-4} cm. dispersed in any medium constitute what we term a colloidal system. In true solution the size of solute particles in solution is upto 1×10^{-7} cm. A colloidal system is always heterogenous and consists of at least two phases: the dispersed phase (the phase constituting the colloidal particles) and the dispersion medium (the medium in which these particles are dispersed).

There are eight types of colloidal solutions possible depending upon the three states of matter, viz, solid, liquid and gases. Gas in colloidal solution is not possible because gases always form homogenous mixture while all the other possible types have been actually obtained. Colloidal solutions are often called sols. A few examples of each type of colloidal system are given in the Table 7.3.

Table 7.3. Some common colloidal systems

Dispersed phase	Dispersion medium	Examples
Gas	Liquid	Foam, whipped cream
Gas	Solid	Pumice stone, bread, rubber
Liquid	Gas	Fog, clouds, insecticide spray
Liquid	Liquid	Milk, emulsified oils and medicines
Liquid	Solid	Cheese, butter, boot polish
Soild	Gas	Smoke, dust storm
Solid	Liquid	Mosit paints, starch dispersed in water, gold, sol. muddy water.
Soild	Solid	Black diamonds, minerals, rubby, glass, gem stone.

Based on the nature of dispersion media, colloids are sometimes grouped as hydrosols (in water), alcohols (in alcohol), benzosols (in benzene), aerosols (in air), etc.

Based upon the mode of preparation of the colloidal solution, different substances may be divided into two categories:

(i) Lyophilic (solvent loving): These are substances like gelatin, gum, starch which readily pass into colloidal solution on simply warming or shaking with a suitable solvent. The solution obtained are very stable and are referred to as reversible colloids since the residue lift after evaporating the dispersion medium again passes into colloidal state on the addition of the solvent.

(ii) Lyophobic (solvent hating): These are substances like metals, their sulphides, oxides etc. which do not form colloidal solutions readily. The colloidal solution can be obtained only by applying special methods. The resulting solution are not very stable and are termed irreversible colloids. They need stabilizing agents to preserve them.

If water is the dispersium medium, the terms used are hydrophilic and hydrophobic sols respectively. Some of the important characteristic of lyophilic and lyophobic colloids are given in a tabular formly Table 7.4.

Table 7.4

Lyophilic Colloids	Lyophobic Colloids
1. Self stabilized	Small quantity of electrolyte is required for stabilization
2. Reversible	Ir-reversible
3. Prepared by simple solution method	Prepared by indirect methods.
4. Mostly organic materials, eg. starch, protens, gums etc.	These are generally inorganic materials i.e. metals, sulphides and oxide sol
5. Large quantity of electrolyte causes coagulation	Even small quantity of electrolyte causes coagulation.
6. Tyndall effect is less distinct	They exhibt Tyndall effect.
7. The particles are not easily detected even under ultra-microscope	The particles are easily detected under ultra-microscope.

Preparation of colloids

Physical methods:

1. *By exchange of solvent*

   Colloidal solutions of substances which are soluble in alcohol but practically insoluble in water (e.g., sulphur and phosphorous) can be obtained by pouring their alcoholic solutions in water. The sols obtained is freed from alcohol by dialysis.

2. *By Grinding*

   The substance to be dispersed is suspended as a course precipitate in the dispersion medium which is then passed through a colloidal mill. A colloidal mill consists of two discs closely held together. The discs roate at a very high speed of about 700 rotations per minute in opposite directions. The method is used to prepare colloidal solutions of sulphur, indigo, aniline blue, paints etc.

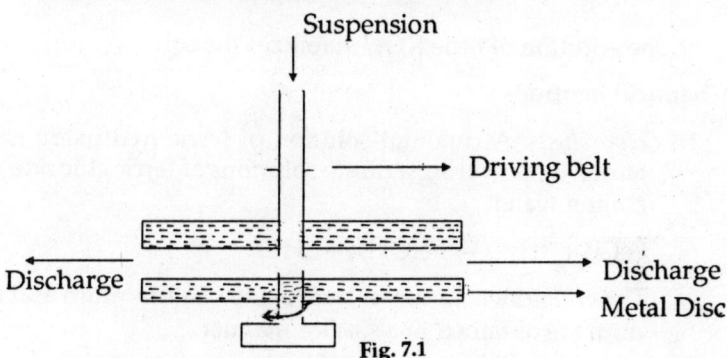

Fig. 7.1

The colloidal solution so formed is stabilized by a protective colloid like gum arabic, tanin etc.

3. *Change of physical state:*

   Colloidal solutions of certain elements are obtained by passing their vapours into cold water containing ammonium chloride or citrate as stabilizer. For example, a sulphur or mercury soil is prepared by boiling sulphur or mercury and then passing the vapours through cold water containing ammonium citrate as stabilizer.

4. *Bredig's Method:*

   This method is used to prepare colloidal solution of metals such as platinum, silver or gold.

Two electrodes of the metal whose colloidal solution is to be prepared are immeresed in dispersion medium such as water. The dispersion medium is kept cooled by sorrounding it with a freezing mixture. An electric arc is struck between the electrodes. As a result, tiny particles break away from the electrodes and get dispersed in the dispersion medium.

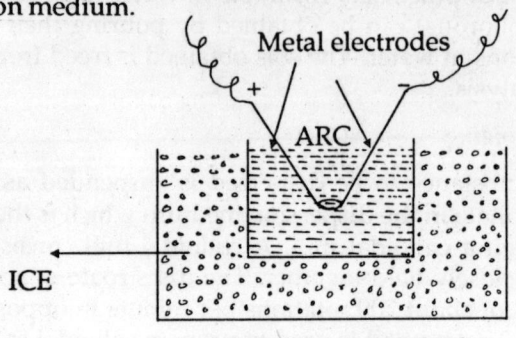

Bredig's arc method

Fig. 7.2

The addition of little KOH stabilizes the sol.

Chemical methods

1. *Hydrolysis:* A colloidal solution of ferric hydroxide is obtained by powering a dilute solutions of ferric chloride into boiling water.

    $$FeCl_3 + 3H_2O \rightarrow Fe(OH)_3 + 3HCl$$

    The colloidal solution of hydroxide of aluminium and thorium are obtained in a similar manner.

2. *Double decomposition:* A colloidal solution of arsenious sulphide is obtained by passing H_2S through a solution of As_2O_3

    $$AS_2O_3 + 3H_2S \rightarrow AS_2S_3 + 3H_2O$$

3. *Oxidation:* A colloidal solution of sulphur is obtained when H_2S is bubbled through an oxidising agent like Br_2 water or dil HNO_3 solution.

    $$H_2S + Br_2 \rightarrow 2HBr + S$$

    $$H_2S + 2HNO_3 \rightarrow 2H_2O + 2NO_2 + S$$

    colloidal solution of iodine is obtained by oxidising HI with HIO_3.

$$5HI + HIO_3 \rightarrow 3H_2O + 3I_2$$

4. *Reduction:* Colloidal solutions of metals like Au, Ag, Pt, Bi etc. can be obtained by reduction of their water soluble compounds using suitable reducing agent like formaldehyde, tannin, stannous chloride. A gold sol is formed on reduction of $AuCl_3$ by $SnCl_2$.

$$2AuCl_3 + 3SnCl_2 \rightarrow 3\ SnCl_4 + 2Au$$

Purification of colloidal solutions

1. Dialysis: is the process of seperating colloidal solutions from true solutions. The apparatus used for carrying out dialysis is called dialyser. Colloidal particles are retained by porous membrane, e.g. parchment bag while crystalloids pass through. Thus colloidal solution can be purified by enclosing it in a parchment bag and placing in running water. Crystalloids present as impurity pass out through the parchment membrane leaving pure sol behind. The process is accelerated to some extent by using hot water in place of cold water (hot dialysis).

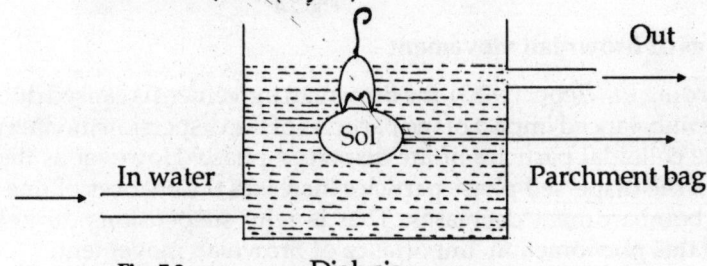

Fig. 7.3   Dialysis

2. Electro-dialysis: In this process electrodes are placed outside the membrane enclosing the colloidal solution. The current is switched on. Then the ions present in the sol tend to migrate towards the oppositely charged electrodes. Consequently the process of dialysis is speeded up and is known as electro-dialysis.

Properties of Colloidal Solutions

Mechanical Properties

1. *Brownian Movement:* Colloidal particles are found to be in continual motion in zig-zag paths when seen under an ultra-microscope. This motion is called Brownian movement. Dust particles floating in air in a dark room constitute

a colloidal solution. When a beam of light is passed through the dark room the dancing of dust particles in the beam of light which becomes visible is an example of Brownian movement.

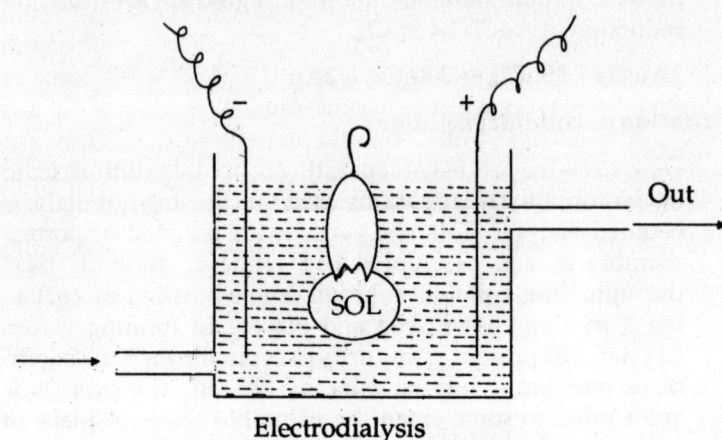

Electrodialysis

Fig. 7.4

Causes of Brownian movement

According to Wiener (1863), the Brownian movement is caused due to the unbalanced impact of the particles of the dispersion medium on the colloidal particles of the dispersed phase. However as the size of the dispersed phase particles increases the chances of unequal bombardment decreases. That is why suspensions do not show this phenomenon. Importance of Brownian movement:

   (i)   Confirmation of Kinetic movement: Brownian movement is an excelent proof of ceaseless motion of molecules just as postulated by kinetic theory.

   (ii)   *Stability of colloidal solutions:* Brownian movement counter acts the force of gravity acting on the colloidal particles. Consequently it is responsible to some extent for the stability of colloidal solution.

  2.   *Diffusion:* Colloidal particles diffuse from a region of higher concentration to another of lower concentration. Their motion being slower than molecules in a true solution, the rate of diffusion is low. This process can be used to seperate colloids of different sizes and also to determine their sizes.

  3.   *Sedimentation:* Colloidal particles tend to settle down very slowly under the influence of gravity. The rate of sedimen-

tation can be increased to a large extent by the use of a high speed centrifuge known as ultracentrifuge.

Electrical properties

4. *Electrical charge:* Lyophobic colloids are electrically charged while lyophilic colloids become electrically charged in the presence of an electrolyte. Colloidal particles carry either positive or negative charges and all the particles of a given colloidal solution carry the same kind of charge. For example $Fe(OH)_3$ sol is positively charged while colloidal AS_2S_3 sol is negatively charged.

5. *Cataphoresis:* In an electric field, the particles of colloidal solution being positively charged, move towards an opposite charged electrode. The movement of colloidal particles under influence of an applied electric field is called electrophoresis or cataphoresis, shown in the Figure.

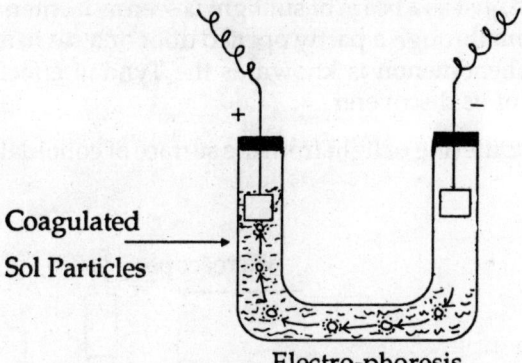

Coagulated Sol Particles →

Fig. 7.5 Electro-phoresis

6. *Electro-Osmosis:* The movement of the dispersion medium under the influence of an electric field when the particles of dispersed phase are prevented from moving is referred to as electro-osmosis. This is demonstrated by the following experiment.

When a potential difference is applied across the electrodes held close to the membrane in compartments B and C, the water begins to move. If the particles carry positive charge, the water will carry negative charge and hence will start moving towards anode and hence the level of water in the side tube T would have been seen to rise. If particles carry negative charge, water will now carry positive charge and the level of water in the side tube T' would start rising.

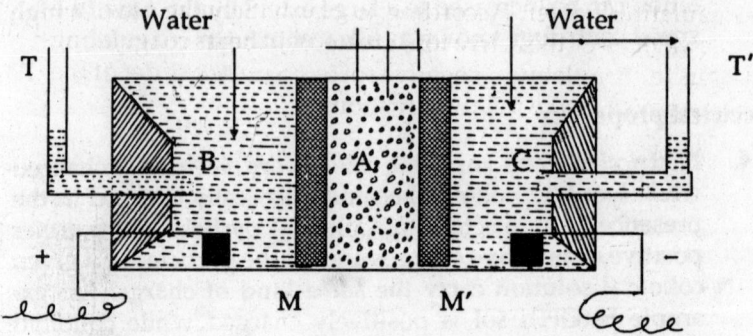

A colloidal system, B and C filled with water, M & M' dialysis membrane.

Fig. 7.6

7. *Optical properties:*

Tyndall Effect (1869) when a beam of light is passed through a true solution, the path of beam through the solution is not visible. But, if the light is passed through the sol, its path becomes visible, just as a beam of sunlight is seen as it enters a darkened room through a partly opened door or a slit in a curtain. This phenomenon is known as the Tyndall effect after the name of its discoverer.

It is due to the scattering of light from the surface of colloidal particles.

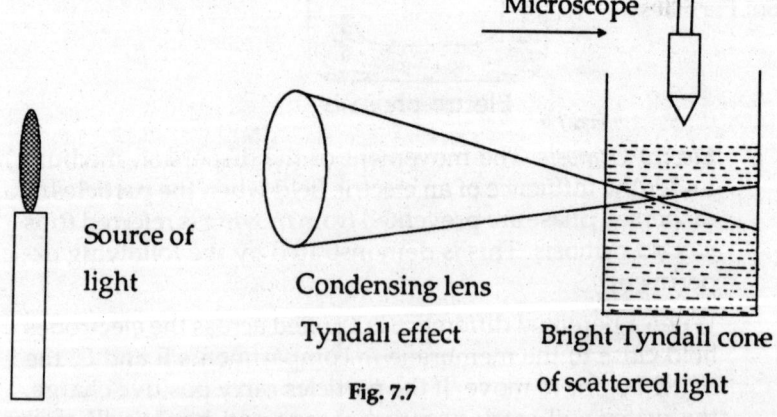

Fig. 7.7

Coagulation of Colloids

A colloidal solution gets precipitated or coagulated by the addition of a suitable electrolyte to it. The coagulation is, in fact, caused by the charge on the ions. Thus, greater the ionic charge, greater will be its coagulating power. According to Hardy Schulze Law, the greater the valency of the active ion, greater will be its coagulating power. Thus to coagulating a negative sol of AS_2S_3, the order of the coagulating power of the following cations is:

$$Al^{3+} > Mg^{2+} > Na^+$$

Similarly to effect the coagulation of a positively charge sol such as $Fe(OH)_3$, the coagulating power of the following anions are arranged as:

$$PO_4^{3-} > SO_4^{2-} > Cl^-$$

The minimum concentration of an electrolyte in milli moles per litre of mixed solution required to cause coagulation of a particular sol is called coagulation or precipitation value of the electrolyte for the sol.

Other factors governing coagulation:

    (i) *Nature of colloid:* Lyophilic colloids are more difficult to coagulate than lyophobic colloids.

    (ii) *Rise of temperature:* Increase in temperature helps in the precipitation e.g. white of an egg gets coagulated on heating.

    (iii) *Centrifuging:* Due to difference in the density of the dispersion medium and the dispersed phase, centrifugation causes coagulation.

    (iv) *Mutual coagulation:* Certain lyophobic colloids cause mutual coagulation on being mixed together. This occurs mainly due to neutrilization of electrical charges of opposite kind. For example, when negatively charged arsenic sulphide sol is added to a positively charged ferric hydroxide sol, in suitable preportions, precipitations of both the sols takes place simultaneously.

    and

    (v) Coagulation can also be brought about by passing an electric current through the sol.

Protective Colloids

Colloidal solution such as those of metals like gold, silver etc can be easily precipitated by addition of a small amount of electrolyte. This can be prevented or retarded by previous addition of a more stable hydrophilic colloids like gelatin, albumin etc. For example, if a small amouunt of gelatin is added to gold sol, it is no longer precipitated by the addition of sodium chloride. This process by which the sol particles are protected from precipitation by electrolytes due to previous addition of some hydrophilic colloids is called protection. The colloid which is added to achieve such a protection is called protective colloid. Other examples of protective colloids are gum, starch. Possibly the potective colloids form a protective coating which covers the particles of lyophobic colloids and this prevents their coagulation.

Lyophilic collids differ in their protective powers Zsig-mondy introduced the term gold number to measure the protective powers of different emulsoids. Gold number is defined as the number of milligrams of protective colloid which prevents the coagulation of 10 ml of a red gold sol on the addition of 1 ml of a 10% solution of sodium chloride.

It has been observed that smaller the value of the gold number, greater will be the protecting power of the protective colloid. Thus out of gelatin, egg albumin, starch, dextrin. Gelatin and egg albumin are the best protective colloids.

Various applications of colloids

1. *Purification of water:* The addition of electrolyte like alum (furnishes Al^{3+}) to impure water coagulates the negatively charged particles of very fine clay. The pure water is decanted off.

2. *Cleansing action of soap:* soap form a colloidal solution when dissolved in water. It removes the dust particles from the cloth by adsorption or by emulsifying the greasy particles sticking to the fabric. This action releases the dirt when washed with water.

3. *Photography:* The photographic films or plates are made by coating the cellulose film or thin glass plates with a colloidal solution of silver bromide in gelatin.

4. *Formation of deltas:* The river water carries in suspended form charged particles of clay, sand etc. On meeting the sea water, the suspended particles of river water are coagulated by the electrolytes (Na^+, K^+, Mg^{2+} ions) present in the sea water.

5. *Rubber industry:* The negatively charged particles of rubber in latex are made to deposit on to wires or handles of various tools (in order to insulate them) by electrophoresis. The article to be rubber plated is made the anode.

6. *Tanning of lather:* Skins and hides are colloidal in character. When hides are soaked in a solution of tannin, the positively charged particles of hide and negatively charged particles of tannin undergo mutual coagulation. This process called tanning, gives hardness to lather.

7. *Smoke precipitations:* Colloidal carbon particles in chimney gases are removed by passing them between high voltage plates. Thi is made use of in Cottrell smoke precipitator.

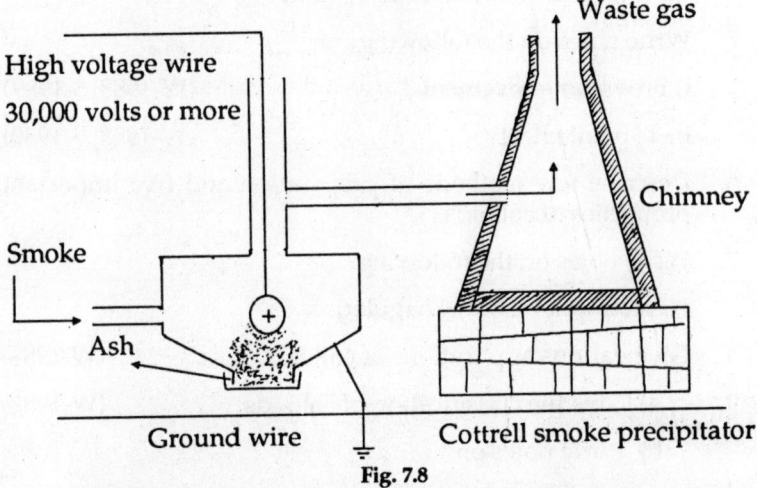

Fig. 7.8

8. *Purification of sugar:* The purification of sugar juice is based on the adsorption of colouring matter by activated charcoal which is colloidal in nature.

9. *Dyeing:* mordants used in dyeing adsorbs the dyes.

10. *Smoke screens:* Smoke screens generally consist of very fine praticles of titanium oxide dispersed in air and are ejected from aeroplanes. They are used in warfare for the purpose of concealment and camouflage.

11. *Sewage disposal:* Sewage contains negatively charged dirt particles. Therefore, sewage on electrophoresis deposits dirt particles at the anode, which may be used as a fertilizer.

QUESTIONS

1. What are the characteristic of colloidal solution? In what respect does a colloidal solution differ from a true solution?

2. Describe any one method for preparation of colloidal solution (W-1989)

3. Write notes on the following:

   i) Dialysis ii) Lyophobic and iii) Lyophilic colloids

4. a. Discuss the characteristic of colloidal solutions.

   b. How are the colloidal solutions of the following prepared:

   i) Arsenious sulphide ii) Gold

5. Write notes on the following:

   i) Brownian movement   (W-1988, S-1989)

   ii) Tyndall effect   (W-1988, S-1989)

6. Describe few methods of preparation and five important properties of colloids.

7. Write notes on the following:

   i) Electrophoresis ii) Coagulation

8. Give various applications of colloids.   (W-1988)

9. a) Give the classification of colloids.   (W-1988)

   b) Write notes on:

   i) Electro Osmosis   (W-1989)

10. a) What is meant by electrophoresis. Give one experiment to illustrate it.

    b) Explain the following:

    i) Formation of Delta ii) Smoke screen

    iii) Rubber platingiv) Sewage disposal

11. Describe in detail various methods employed for the preparation of colloids.   (S-1989)

12. What do you understand be the term "Electrophoresis"? How would you demonstrate this phenomenon.   (S-1989)

13. a) Discuss the important properties of colloidal system

    b) Differentiate the following:
    i) Colloidal solution and true solution
    ii) Colloidal dispersion and polymer solution (S-1990)

OBJECTIVE TYPE QUESTIONS

14. Fill in the blanks with the appropriate word/words:

    (i) The process for purifying a colloidal solution by placing it in a parchment bag kept in water is called ---------.

    (ii) If the dispersed phase has affinity for the dispersion medium, the colloid is known as --------------------.

    (iii) Colloidal particles are found to be in a state of rapid irregular motion known as -------------------------.

    (iv) Migration of colloidal particles under the influence of an electric field is called -------------------------.

    (v) Colloidal particles are not visible under a microscope but can be seen as points of light with the help of -------------- due to -------------.

    (vi) Colloidal solutions are generally purified by ------------.

    (vii) If the dispersed phase has hatred for the dispersium medium, the colloid is known as --------------.

    (viii) A colloidal solution essentially consists of ------------ phases namely ---------- and ---------.

    (ix) Colloids are essentially -------- and not a class of substances

    (x) The phenomenon of precipitation of a colloidal sols by the addition of an electrolyte is known as ---------------.

15. Choose the correct answer to the following:

    (i) The size of the colloidal paraticles ranges between 10^{-3} cm to 10^{-5} cm/10^{-4} cm to 10^{-7} cm.

    (ii) The random or zig-zag motion of the colloidal particles in the dispersed medium is refered to as: Brown-ian movement/Tyndall effect.

    (iii) The presence of electric charge on the colloidal particles is indicated by Electrolysis/Electrophoresis.

    (iv) The process of a seperation of crystalloids by using a semipermeable membrane is refered as Filtration/Dialysis.

    (v) How many phases are present in a colloidal system Two/Four.

(vi) Blood contains negatively charged/positevely charged particles

(vii) Colloidal particles are visible to the naked eye/under an ultramicroscope.

(viii) The coagulation power of Fe^{3+} is higher/lower than Ba^{2+}.

(ix) Alum purifies muddy water by dialysis/coagulation.

(x) When the dispersion medium in a colloidal system is taken as gas it is referred to as Hydrosol/Aerosol.

ANSWERS

14. i) Dialysis, ii) Lyophilic, iii) Brownian movement, iv) Electrophoresis v) Ultra-microscope, scattering of light (Tyndall effect), vi) Dialysis, vii) Lyophobic, viii) Two, dispersed phase, dispersion medium, ix) A state of matter, x) Coagulation.

15. i) 10^{-4} cm to 10^{-7} cm, ii) Brownian movement, iii) Electrophoresis, iv) Dialysis, v) Two, vi) negatively, vii) ultra-microscope, viii) higher, ix) coagulation, x) Aerosol.

Chapter VIII

Principles and Methods of Purification of Substances

Crystalline and Amorphous substances

Solid exist in either crystalline or amorphous state, crystalline substances have a definite regid shapes. Every crystal is contained within a well defined set of surfaces which are called planes. It has a sharp melting point and a definite three dimensional arrangement of constituent particles. When we try to cut a crystalline solid with a sharp edged tool it gives a clean cleavage, but an amorphous substance gives an irregular or conchoidal fracture. Amorphous solids include substances like glass, fused silica, rubber and polymer of high molecular masses.

Crystalline solids may be further classified according to the nature of the particles constituting them and the binding forces between them. We have the following types of crystalline solid.

(1) *Ionic solids:* Network of positive and negative ions systematically arranged held together by strong forces of electro-static attraction. They are brittle, have high m.p., are poor conductors of electricity and heat. They have very high heats of fusion. They are generally soluble in water and insoluble in non-polar solvents, such as Carbon tetra-chloride and benzene:

Examples: Salts like LiF, NaCl, KCl, KNO_3 etc.

(ii) *Molecular solids:* The constitutents consists of small molecule held together by weak Vander Waals forces. They are soft and have low m.p. they vaporise very readily, have low heats of fusion. They are electrical insulators and poor thermal conductors. They have usually, very low solubility in polar solvents like water.

Examples: Solid CO_2, solid methane, Wax, Iodine, Sulphur, etc.

(iii) *Covalent solids:* A net work of chemically bound atoms of one or more kinds held together by covalent bond forces. They are very hard, have high m.p., poor conductors of heat and electricity and have high heats of fusion.

Examples: Diamond, Graphite, Silicon, Quartz etc.

(iv) *Metallic solids:* Positive ions in a sea of electrons held together by electrical attraction. They are very soft to very hard, have low to very high m.p. They are good conductors of heat and electricity, have metallic lustre. They are malleable and ductile and have moderate heats of fusion. Examples: Common metals and some alloys.

Criteria of Purity

Melting point and boiling point: Melting point of a crystalline solid is the temperature at which the solid begins to change into a liquid under a pressure of one atmosphere. For pure substances, the change from solid to the liquid state is quite sharp (within 0.5°) hence the temperature is valuable for purposes of identification. Experimental Determination of the Melting point.

The apparatus employed for the determination of the melting point of a given solid is shown in the lFig. 8.1 the finely powdered and

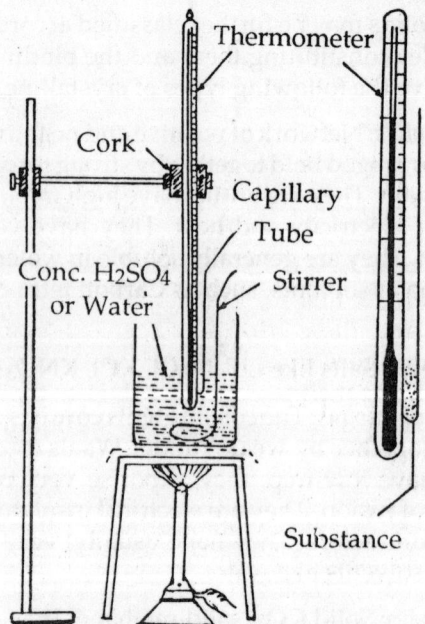

Fig. 8.1. Determination of melting point.

carefully dried substance is charged into a capillary tube sealed at one end. The capillary tube is wetted with the liquid in the beaker and placed alongside a thermometer fixed in an iron stand in such a way that the substance in it is at the same level as the middle of the bulb of the thermometer. The thermometer is now lowered in a beaker containing sulphuric acid (b.p. 338°C) . The beaker is heated slowly and the temperature of the both kept uniform by gently but constant stirring with a glass rod. The temperature at which the substance just melts and becomes transparent is recorded. The sulphuric acid bath can be replaced by water-bath for melting points below 100°C.

Boiling Point: is a fixed temperature at which a liquid begins to boil or the temperature at which the vapour pressure of a liquid becomes equal to the atmosphere pressure. The normal boiling point is a characteristic property of a liquid.

Experimental determination of the boiling point -

(i) Distillation method if enough liquid is available, its boiling point is determined in a ordinary distillation apparatus. (Fig. 8.3). A pure liquid will distil at a constant temperature which is its boiling point. In case the liquid is impure, the boiling point will rise during distillation.

(ii) *Siwoloboff's method (1886):*

This method is employed were only a small quantity of the liquid are available. The apparatus used is shown in Fig. 8.2. A few drops of the liquid are placed in the small thin-walled test tube, attached to the thermometer by means of a rubber band. A capillary tube, sealed about 1 cm. from the lower end, is placed in the test tube which is then heated in a bath containing water or sulphuric acid (any liquid whose boiling point is higher than of the substance under investigation). The bath liquid stirred continuously with a ring stirrer. At first air bubbles rise from the lower end of the capillary and these become more and more numerous as the temperature goes up. The burner is then removed and stirring continued. The thermometer is read when the evolution of bubbles just stops. This is the boiling point of the liquid under examination.

Crystallisation

This is most common method used for the purification of solid organic substances. In this process, the crystals of a pure substance are obtained by cooling its hot saturated solution in a suitable solvent. In actual practice, the impure organic substance is dis-

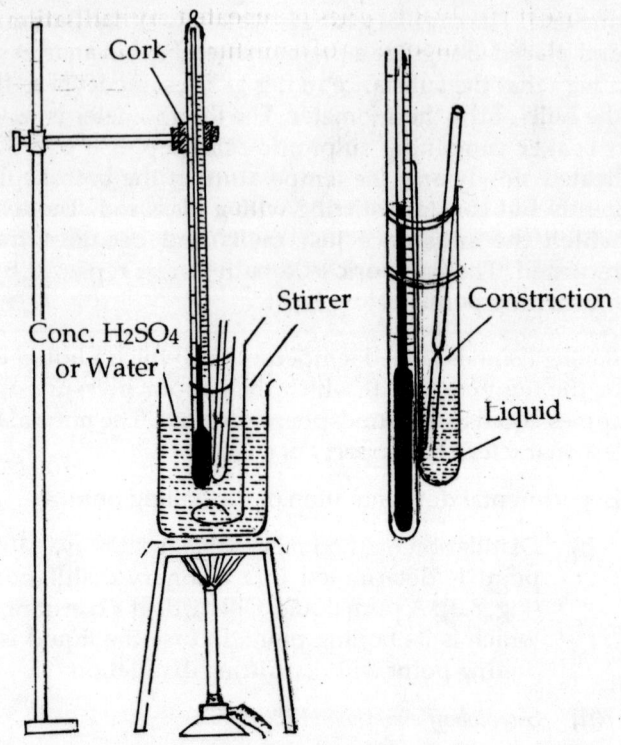

Fig. 8.2. Determination of boiling point.

solved in a minimum quantity of hot solvent so as to obtain a saturated solution. It is dicolorised with bone charcoal if necessary and filtered while hot. The filtrate on being allowed to cool slowly in a shallow dish deposits crystals of the pure substance. These are dried by pressing between folds of filter paper or by using a porous plate. The crystals are finally dried in a vacuum dessicator.

Fractional Crystallisation

This method is used in the separation of two organic solids which have quite different solubilities in the same solvent. The saturated solution containing the mixture of two compounds which do not have large difference in their solubilities is cooled as usual. On cooling, the less soluble constitutent of the mixture separate out first and may be contaminated with a little more soluble substance. The mother liquor is now very rich in the more soluble substance and on further concentration and cooling will yield the crystals of more soluble substance contaminated with less soluble substance. The process is repeated several times to get the pure crystals of the two substances. This process is called fractional crystallisation because it involves a series of repeated crystallisation in order to seperate the components of a mixture.

Purification of Liquids

Distillation: It is the process of converting a liquid into vapour, condensing the vapours on cooling back to liquid. It is used for seperating an organic liquid (Which does not decompose on boiling) from non volatile impurities.

The apparatus used for distillation is shown in Fig. 8.3 it consists of a distillation flask fitted with a thermometer in its neck and a Leibig's condenser at the side tube. The liquid to be purified is

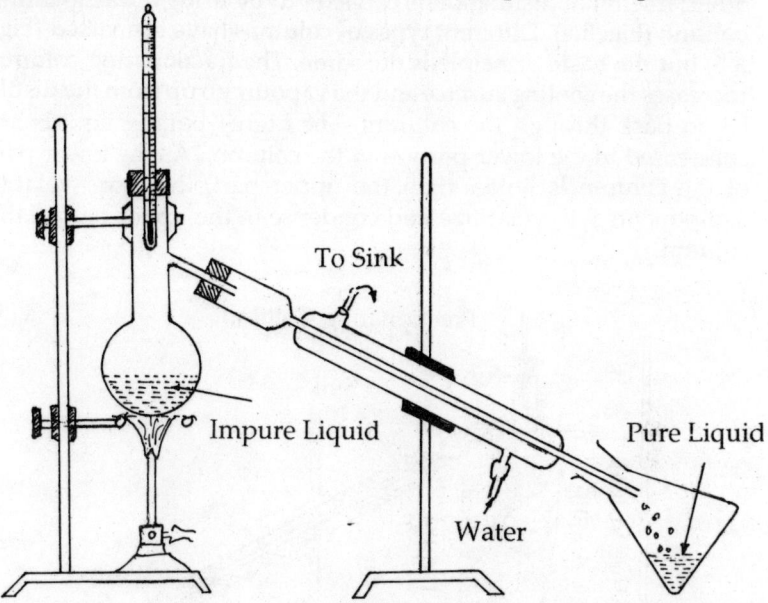

To Sink

Impure Liquid

Pure Liquid

Water

Fig. 8.3. Distillation.

placed in the distillation flask and the thermometer so adjusted that its bulb stands just below the opening into the side tube. A receiver is attached to the lower end of the condenser to collect the condensed liquid. On heating the distillation flask, the thermometer first records a rise in temperature which soon becomes constant. At this point, which is boiling point of the liquid, most of the liquid passes over and is collected in the receiver. The non-volatile impurities are left behind in the flask. Towards the end of the process, temperature rises once again. The distillation is stopped at this stage and receiver disconnected.

If the boiling point of the liquid to be distilled is higher than 373k, the water condenser is replaced by air - condenser. A few pieces of unglazed porcelain are added in the distillation flask to prevent bumping. While distilling highly volatile and inflammable liquid such as ether, the distillation flask is heated on a hot plate. In case of high boiling liquids the flask is heated directly with the flame.

Distillation can be used to seperate ether (boiling at 308k) or petroleum ether (boiling between 313 and 333k) from other liquids boiling above 370k (e.g. toluene boiling at 383k).

Fractional Distillation

If the boiling points of the liquids to be seperated are close to each other, fractional distillation is carried out by using a fractionating column (Fig. 8.4). Different types of columns have been used (Fig. 8.5) but the basic principle is the same. The fractionating column increases the cooling surface and the vapours go up from the distillation flask through the column., The higher boiling liquids are condensed in the lower portion of the column. As the lower part of the column is hotter than the upper part, the more volatile components will volatilize and condense in the upper part of the column.

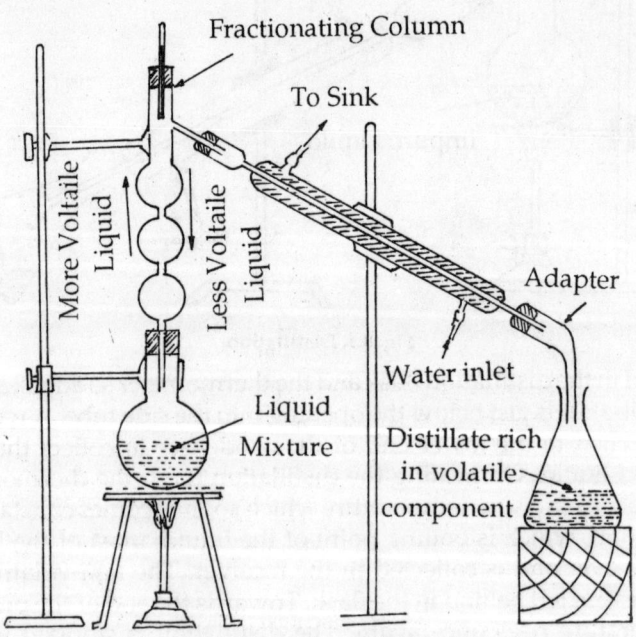

Fig. 8.4. Fractional Distillation.

Fractional distillation has been found very useful in the separation of various fractions of petroleum, coal tar and crude alcohol.

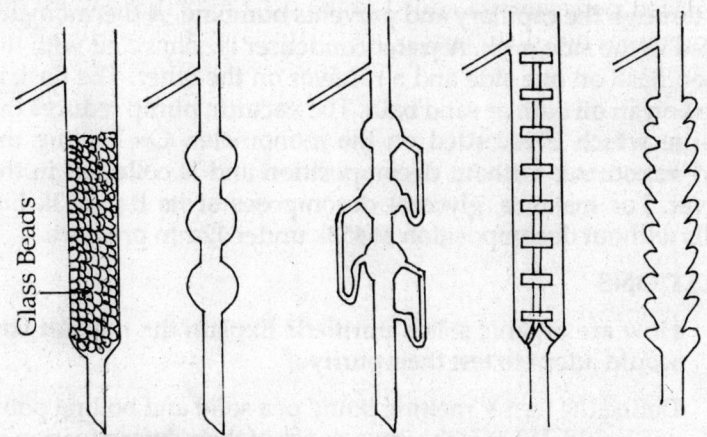

Fig. 8.5. Different types of fractionating columns.

Distillation under reduced pressure

High boiling liquids as well as liquids which decompose at or below their normal boiling points are generally distilled at lower temperature under reduced pressure (Fig. 8.6) by creating a partial vacuum inside the apparatus.

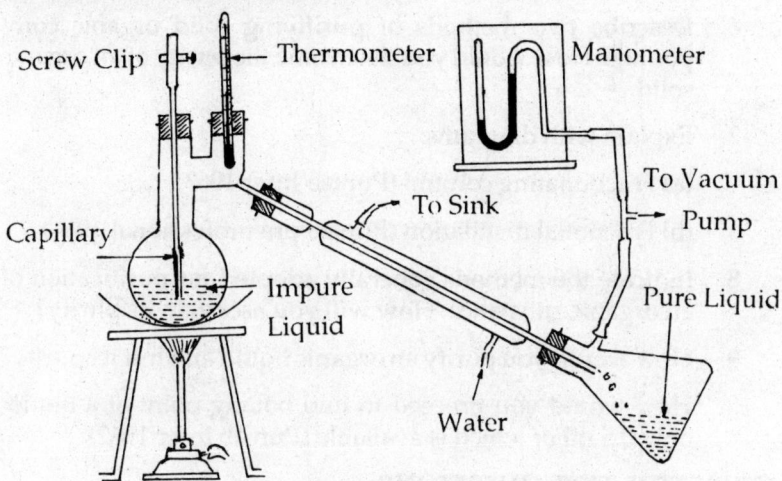

Fig. 8.6. Distillation under reduced pressure.

The apparatus consists of a Claisen's flask fitted with a long capillary tube in the main neck. During distillation a stream of bubbles rises through the capillary and prevents bumbing. A thermometer is fitted in the side neck. A water condenser is connected with the Claisen flask on one side and a receiver on the other. The flask is heated on an oil bath or sand bath. The vacuum pump reduces the pressure which is recorded on the monometer. On heating the liquid vapourises without decomposition and is collected in the receiver. For instance, glycerol decomposes at its b.p. 563k but distills without decomposition at 453k under 12mm pressure.

QUESTIONS

1. How are organic solids purified? Explain the method you would adopt to test their purity.

2. Define the terms 'melting point' of a solid and boiling point of a liquid. What is the importance of their determination in Organic chemistry?

3. Name two methods of purification of Organic compounds.

4. Write short note on:

   (a) Crystallisation   (b) Distillation

5. Explain briefly with the help of diagram "Vacuum distillation".

6. Describe two methods of purifiying solid organic compounds. How would you determine the purity of an organic solid.

7. Explain with diagrams:

   (a) Fractionating column (Punjab Inter 1963)

   (b) Fractional distillation (Punjab pre professional 1964)

8. Indicate the methods generally adopted for purification of an organic substance. How will you ascertain its purity?

9. How would you purify an organic liquid and test its purity?

10. How would you proceed to find boiling point of a liquid, only 0.5 ml of which is available (Punjab Inter 1962)

OBJECTIVE TYPE QUESTIONS

11. (a) *Fill in the blanks:*

1. The criteria of purity of an organic solid is its------------------.

2. The criteria of purity of an organic liquids is its----------------.

3. The high boiling points liquids are purified by----------------.

4. Purification of organic solid compounds largely depends upon the right choice of the-------------------------.

5. -------------------- is a process in which a liquid is converted into its vapours which on cooling condense to give back the liquid.

6. The temperature at which a solid begins to change into a liquid is called-------------------------.

7. The physical properties used as criteria of purity of organic compounds are -------------------and-------------------------.

(b) *Select the correct answer:*

1. Fractional crystillation is carried out to seperate such mixture

   (i) Organic solids having equal solubilities in a suitable solvent.

   (ii) Organic solids having small difference in their solubilities in suitable solvent.

2. *Filtration is used to seperate*

   i) a mixture of solids ii) a solution from suspended solids.

3. Liquids which decompose below their normal boiling points can be distilled at low temperature by

   i) increasing the pressure ii) decreasing the pressure

4. Seperation of petroleum into different fractions is done by

   i) filtration ii) fractional distillation

ANSWERS

(a) 1. Sharp melting point 2. Sharp boiling point 3. Distillation under reduced pressure 4. Solvent 5. Distillation 6. Melting point 7. Melting point, Boiling point

(b) 1. (ii)

    2. (ii)

    3. (ii)

    4. (ii)

Chapter IX

Fuels

A combustible material which on burning produces heat energy without the production of undesirable by-products is called a fuel.

Classification of fuels and their chemical composition:

Fuel can be classified in three ways:

(a) As solid, liquid and gaseous depending upon their state of aggregation e.g.,

Solid fuels: Wood, peat, lignite, butuminous and anthracite coal.

Liquid fuels: Petroleum

Gaseous fuel: Natural gas.

(b) Fuels can be classified as natural fuels and processed fuels e.g.,

Natural fuels: Wood, coal, petroleum, natural gas

Processed fuels: Charcoal, coke, petrol, kerosene oil, diesel oil, water gas and coal gas etc.

(c) Another classification distinguishes fuels as primary and secondary e.g.,

Primary fuels: Coal, wood, and petroleum are used directly to produce heat.

Secondary fuels: are derived from primary fuels. Coal gas, water gas and producer gas are examples of secondary fuels.

Chemical composition

A. *Natural solid fuels*

Wood   Air dired wood contains 15% moisture carbon about 50%

Coal	It is largely used as domestic fuel. The successive stage in the transformation of vegetable matter into coal are:

Wood → peat → lignite → bituminous

Coal → anthracite coal

The following are the kinds of coal in use:

(i) *Peat:* Air dried peat is carbon 60%. Peat is not a good fuel.

(ii) *Lignite:* Air dried lignite contains carbon 60 - 70%

(iii) *Bituminous coal:* carbon is about 80%

(iv) *Anthracite:* carbon content about 90%.

In general coal obtained from coal mines is a mixture of complex carbon compounds and free carbon.

B. *Natural liquid fuels:*

Petroleum	Composition varies from one oil field to another. It consists mainly of aliphatic hydrocarbon, cyclo paraffin and hydrocarbon of the aeromatic series with only small quantity of nitrogen, oxygen or sulphur containing compounds. Carbon 79 to 87%.

C. *Natural Gaseous fuels:*

Natural gas	Source petroleum fields. It contains mainly methane. Used for domestic purposes and in industry.

Processed Fuels

A. Solid fuels:

Wood charcoal:	It is obtained from wood and is essentially composed of carbon 70% and rest is ash and other impurities.
Coke:	It is obtained from Bituminous coal by destructive distillation. It is composed of primarily free carbon.

B. Liquid fuels:

(i) Gasoline:

C_7 - C_{12} composition range. It is suitable fuel for automobiles and aeroplanes.

(ii) Kerosene oil:

C_{12} - C_{15} composition range. It is good fuel for stoves and jet engines..

(iii) Diesel oil:

C_{15} - C_{18} composition range. It is used in diesel engines.

(iv) Methylated spirit:

It is obtained form sugar or starch by fermentation. It contains ethyl alcohol and little methyl alcohol/naphtha

C. *Gaseous fuel:*

(i) Cooking gas (LPG):

It is a mixture of butane and isobutane and is obtained from petroleum.

(ii) Bio gas:

Composition methane, carbon dioxide, hydrogen, hydrogen sulphide. It is 65% methane, which is an excellent fuel. It is obtained from animal and plant wastes.

(iii) Water gas:

It is obtained from coke. It is chiefly a mixture of CO and H_2.

(iv) Producer gas:

It is obtained from coke. It is mixture of CO, H_2, N_2, CO_2 and CH_4.

(v) Coal gas: It is obtained from coal. It is mixture of CO, CO_2, N_2. H_2, CH_4, unsaturated hydrocarbons (C_2H_4, C_2H_2, C_6H_6) and O_2.

(vi) Oil gas: It is obtained by the cracking of Kerosene oil. It is a mixture of CH_4, H_2, CO and CO_2.

Characteristic of a good fuel

The following are the characteristic of a good fuel:

1. It should have a high calorific value.

2. It should have proper ignition temperature.

3. It should have moderate rate of combustion.

4. It should not leave much ash behind.

5. It should not pollute the air on burning.

6. It should be in expensive.

7. It should be available readily and in large quantity.

8. It shold be easy and safe to store.

9. It should be easy and safe to transport.

Calorific values

The quantity of fuel is evaluated from its calorific value. It is defined as the amount of heat obtained upon complete combustion of one gram of fuel. It is expressed in Cal/joule. Higher the calorific value of a fuel the greater is its fuel value.

Experimental determination of calorific value of solid and liquid FUELS

The apparatus used is a bomb calorimeter shown in the Fig. 9.1. The inner vessel or the bomb and its cover are made of strong steel

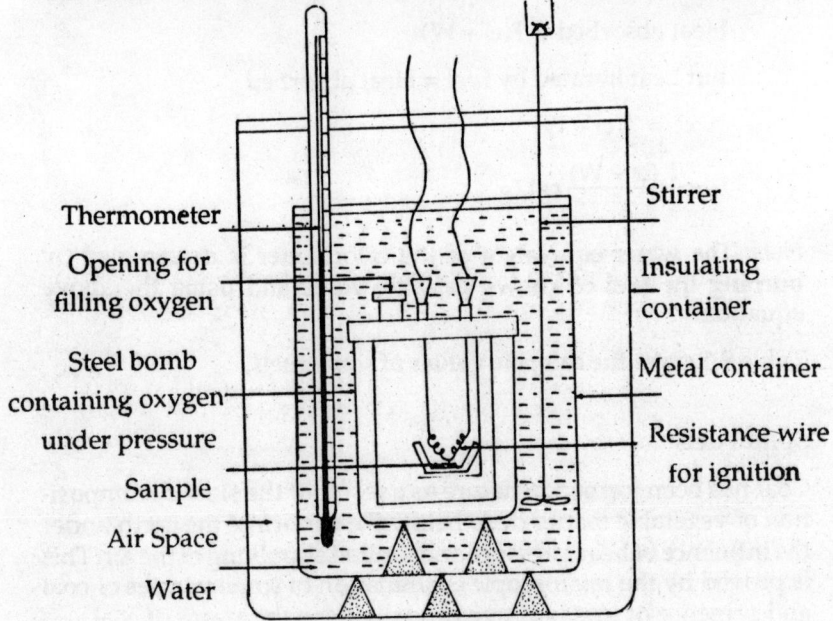

Fig. 9.1. A Bomb calorimeter.

and coated inside with platinum or some other non-oxidisable material. A weighed quantity of the substance is taken in the platinum cup and the bomb is filled with oxygen under a pressure of 20-25 atmosphere and then sealed. The bomb is then lowered in water, placed in a air jacketed and polished metallic calorimeter so as to minimise error due to radiation. It is provided with a stirrer and a sensitive thermometer. The temperature is noted and the reaction is initiated by passing an electric current, through the platinum wire. The rise of temperature of the water in the calorimeter is noted.

Calculations

Let

Mass of the fuel ignited = x gm.

Mass of the water in the calorimeter = ω gm.

Water equivalent of calorimeter = W gm.

Rise in temp. of water and calorimeter = $T^\circ C$

Calorific value of the fuel = L

Heat librated by the burning of the fuel = xL

Heat absorbed = $T(\omega + W)$

But heat librated by fuel = Heat absorbed

$\therefore xL = T(\omega + W)$

$$L = \frac{T(\omega + W)}{x} \text{ cal/g}$$

Note: The water equivalent of the calorimeter is determined by burning the fuel of known calorific value and using the above equation.

Table 9.1 gives the calorific values of some fuels.

Solid Fuels

Coal has been formed in nature as a result of the slow decomposition of vegetable matter deep below the surface of the earth under the influence of heat, pressure and limited supplying of the air. This is proved by the microscopic examination of some varities of coal and presence of fossils of trees and plants in the seams of coal.

Table 9.1

Fuel	Calorific value in kilo joule/g.
Solids	
Coal	25 - 33
Charcoal	33
Liquids	
Kerosene	48
Diesel oil	45
Ethanol	30
Gases	
Hydrogen	150
Methane	55
Butane (LPG)	55

Types of Coal: There are two types,

i) Bituminous coal and ii) Anthracite.

(i) Bituminous coal: It is the common variety of coal. It is black hard stony substance and burns with a smoky flame. It contains about 80% cabon. Cannel coal is another variety of the bituminous coal and burns like a candle.

(ii) Anthracite coal: It is very hard and brittle, has high ignition temperature and does not burn with a smoky flame. It produces very high temperature and contains about 90% carbon. It is final stage in coal formation. Coal is found in India in fairly large amounts in Ranigang (West Bengal) Jharia and Bokaro (Bihar).

Analysis of coal

The elements C, H, S, N, O and ash are estimated as follows:

Ultimate Analysis: This is useful for combustion calculation.

1. **C and H:**

   A small weighed quantity 0.2 g of coal is burnt in a current of oxygen in a combustion apparatus. CO_2 and H_2O formed are absorbed in a weighed potash bulb and calcium chloride tubes. The increase in weight of potash bulb gives the weight of CO_2 formed from cabon in coal. The increase in weight of calcium chloride tubes gives the weight of H_2O formed from H_2 in coal. From the weight of CO_2 and H_2O formed % of C and H is calculated.

2. *S:* present in coal is converted into sulphate in the bomb calorimeter from weighed sample which is precipitated as Barium sulphate, on the addition of Barium chloride solution. The precipitate is filtered, washed and dried. From the weight of barium sulphate, the percentage of S is calculated.

3. *N:* is estimated by taking a small weighed quantity of coal (lg) converting it into ammonium sulphate by heating with concentrated sulphuric acid and K_2SO_4 (catalyst) in Kjeldahl's flask. Ammonium sulphate is heated with sodium hydroxide solution. Ammonia gas evolved is absorbed in a known volume of $N/10$ H_2SO_4. The excess of the acid is determined by the titrating against $N/10$ NaOH. From this the exact volume of H_2SO_4 used in neutralising ammonia is known. From the weight of ammonia librated, the % of N can be calculated.

4. *Ash:* A small weighed quantity of coal is heated to $725°C$ in presence of air. Complete combustion takes place and ash is left behind. The ash is weighed and its % calculated accordingly.

5. *O:* It is obtained by substracting the sum of the five components from 100. Or % oxygen = 100 - % age of (C + H + S + N + Ash) There is no direct method for its estimation.

B. *Proximate Analysis:* It gives information regarding the practical utility of the fuel. It consists in the determination of moisture, volatile matter, fixed carbon and ash in the fuel as under:-

1. *Moisture:* The % of moisture is found by drying a weighed quantity of sample of coal under standard conditions at 377k to 383k.

2. *Volatile matter:* It is determined by heating a dried sample of coal obtained in (1) in a covered crucible for 7 minutes at

1223k. The loss in weight minus the moisture, gives the amount of volatile matter.

3. *Ash:* The % age of ash is determined in the same way as in the ultimate analysis.

4. *Fixed carbon:* It is obtained by subtracting from 100, the % of moisture, volatile matter and ash.

Or 100 - %age of moisture + volatile matter + Ash.

Other varities of coal

Peat   This is the first stage of the conversion of vegetable matter into coal and contains a large percentage of organic matter. Carbon contents is about 60%. It is not a good fuel

Lignite   Is next stage to peat. It is a dark brown substance fairly hard but still contains some unconverted vegetable matter. Carbon content is about 60-70%. It is also not a good fuel because of its low carbon content

Liquid Fuels

Petroleum   (Latin petra = rock and oleum = oil).

                     It is a dark viscous liquid found trapped in certain porous geological strata.

Origin

There are many theories about the origin of petroleum. The present view is that it is of organic in origin and is formed by the decomposition of animal and vegetable matter in the interior of the earth under high pressure and temperature in the presence of little air. This view is supported by the presence of chlorophyll, resins, haemin, optically active compounds of nitrogen and sulphur in peteroleum. It is believed that petroleum orginates from moraine organism.

Some of the leading petroleum producing region are U.S.A, Russia, West Asian countries and Venezuela. In India oil fields are located in Assam, Gujarat and Maharasthra. Recently, we have started getting oil and gas from the high seas off Bombay.

Mining of Petroleum

Petroleum occurs at depths which vary from 300-10,000 feet. It is brought to the surface by drilling wells through the overlying strata into the oil-bearing sand stone (Fig. 9.2).

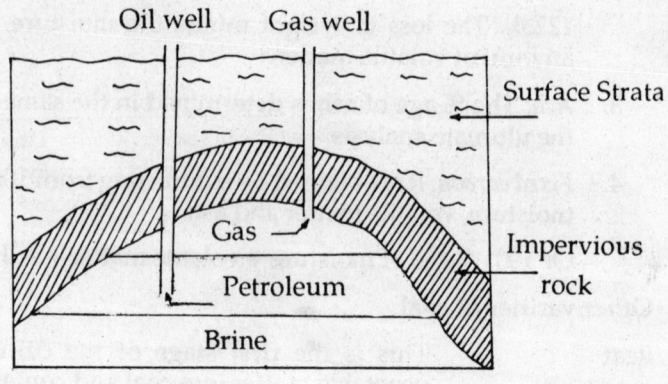

Fig. 9.2. Mining of Petroleum.

When boring is done the oil comes out in a rushing stream due to the pressure of natural gas. When the pressure of gas subsides, it is brought out by pumping. It is taken by means of underground pipes several hundred miles long to the refinary.

Composition of Petroleum

It is essentially a mixture of hydrocarbons of the paraffin series, cycloparaffins and hydrocarbons of the aromatic series. The actual composition, however, varies with the place of origin. It is classified as paraffin base if the crude oil remaining after the removal of volatile hydrocarbons is composed mainly of alkanes and as asphalt base if the residual crude oil is composed of cycloalkanes.

Refining of Petroleum

Crude petroleum is washed with acid and alkali solution to remove the basic and acidic impurities and is then subjected to fractional distillation. Products of typical fractionation of petroleum are given in Table 9.2 with their boiling ranges and uses.

The crude oil is heated to 650k and then flashed into a fractionating column made of steel. The vapours of the oil rise up in the fractionating column become cooler and then condense on the shelves having opening at various heights. The highest boiling fraction condenses at the bottom and the lowest boiling fractions at the top which are continuously removed. The uncondensed gases escape at the head of the column (Fig. 9.3). Several fractions are obtained each one of which is a mixture of hydrocarbons and boils in a certain range of temperature.

Table 9.2

Name	composition	Boiling range 'K'	Uses
Gaseous	C1 - C5	113 - 303	Gaseous fuel, production of carbon black, hydrogen, gasoline.
Petroleum	C5 - C7	303 - 363	Solvent (used in dry-cleaning clothes)
Gasoline	C7- C12	343 - 473	Motor fuel
Kerosene	C12 - C15	448 - 548	Illuminant, fuel
Disel oil	C15 - C18	523 - 673	Fuel for disel engine and cracking
Fuel oil			
Lubricating oil	C16 and up	623 & up	Lubrication
Greases.			
Petroleum-jelly			
Paraffin wax	C20 and up	melts (325 -330)	candles, water proofing fabrics.
Petroleum coke		residue	As fuel. electrodes.

Gasoline obtained by fractional distillation of petroleum is known as straight run, gasoline.

Rating of Fuels

In an internal combustion engine the mixture of fuel vapours and air passes from carburettor to the cylinder and is compressed before

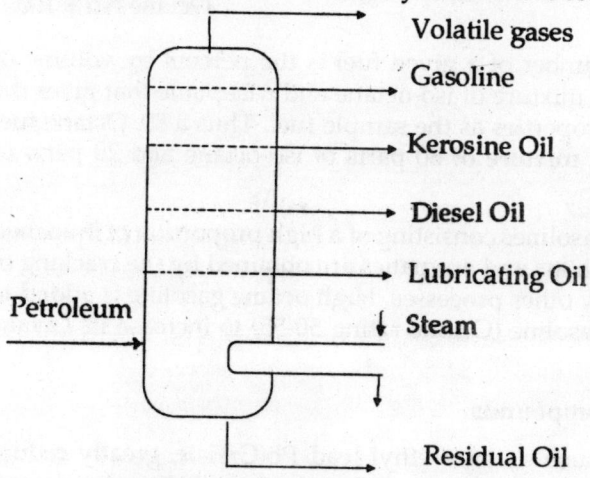

Fig. 9.3. Flow sheet of fractional distillation of crude oil.

ignition. Some hydrocarbons form mixtures with air that detonate on compression, that is before the spark has passed. Pre-ignition of fuel in the cylinder ahead of the flame is called knocking, this decreases the power and causes damage to the cylinder and the piston of the engine. Knocking produces a metallic sound.

The maximum compression which can be achieved without any knocking taking place depends upon the nature of fuel. Thus, it is useful to know the anti-knock value of each fuel.

The anti-knock value of fuel is usually expressed in terms of Octane number (for gasoline) and cetane number (for diesel fuel).

Octane number: n-heptane when used as a fuel is found to lead to too much knocking is assignated an Octane number of zero.

Iso-octane (2, 2, 4- trimethyl pentane)

On the other hand, does not produce knocking to any extent under similar conditions is given a value of 100. This is because, the latter was considered to be an ideal fuel at one time.

$$CH_3. CH_2. CH_2. CH_2. CH_2. CH_2. CH_3$$

n-heptane
Octane No = 0

$$CH_3-CH-CH_2-C-CH_3$$

with CH_3 group on top, and CH_3, CH_3 below

2, 2, 4-trimethyl pentane
(Iso-octane)
Octane No = 100

The Octane number of a given fuel is the percent by volume of iso-octane in a mixture of iso-octane and n-heptane that gives the same knock properties as the sample fuel. Thus a 80. Octane fuel behaves like a mixture of 80 parts of iso-octane and 20 parts of n-heptane.

High octane gasolines consisting of a high proportion of branched chain hydrocabons and aromatics are obtained by the cracking of alkanes and by other processes. High octane gasoline is added to straight-run gasoline (Octane rating 50-55) to increase its Octane rating.

Anti-knock compounds

Compounds such as tetra ethyl lead $Pb(C_2H_5)_4$, greatly reduce knocking and are added upto 0.01% in the gasoline. Lead compounds are poisonous and also contribute to air pollution. Gasoline which contain this additive are known as ethyl or leaded gasoline. Tetra ethyl lead dissociates into ethyl radicals which prevent the explosive burning of the fuel. To prevent the deposition of lead in the cylinder ethylene dibromide is added to the gasoline. It breaks down in the engine to ethylene and bromine. The latter reacts with lead forming lead dibromide which is volatile and is swept from the engine in the exhaust gases.

Tetra ethyl lead $Pb(C_2H_5)_4$ is known as anti-knock compound and was first introduced by Midgley in 1922.

Cetane number

Diesel engines differ from gasoline engines. In case of gasoline engines, fuel air mixture is ignited with the help of a spark from the sparking plug. In the case of diesel engines, the fuel-air mixture is ignited spontaneously by high temperature generated by compression instead of using a spark. Here, air alone is drawn into the cylinder and compressed in the ratio of 14-17 to 1. Due to high compression temperatre rises to about 570k. Diesel is then injected as a fine spray and spontaneous ignition occurs.

For compression ignition engines, straight chain hydrocarbons are superior to branched chain hydrocarbons. Cetane (n-hexadecane $C_{16}H_{34}$) ignites rapidly and is given a rating of 100 where as α-methyl naphthalene ignites slowly and is rated as O.

CH_3

$CH_3\text{-}(CH_2)_{14}\text{-}CH_3$

n-hexadecane
Cetane No = 100

α-methyl naphthalene
Cetane No = 0

Cetane number is the percentage of cetane in the cetane and α-methyl naphthalene mixture which has the same ignition qualities as the sample fuel. Diesel engines have high efficency and use less expensive fuel as compared to engines employing gasoline.

Kerosene Oil: Composition $C_{12} - C_{15}$

Boiling range (k) 448 - 548

Uses: Illuminant; fuel for stoves; for

making oil gas and jet propulsion fuel.

Kerosene oil used in lamps should not be very volatile at ordinaray temperature to form explosive mixtures with air. The lowest temperature at which an oil gives off a sufficient amount of vapour to form an explosive mixture with air is termed its Flash Point. It is determined by "Abel's apparatus".

Laws have been made by different Governments forbidding the sale of oils having flash points below a certain minimum. The minimum flash point prescribed differ in different countries. In India, the flash point is $44^{\circ}C$.

Alcohol

Ethyl alcohol is obtained by the fermentation of sugar or starch. Denatured ethyl alcohol under the name of methylated spirit has been used in stoves and as illuminant.

Ethyl alcohol can be used as a fuel in internal combustion engines. For this purpose there should be no traces of water. Thus absolute alcohol used for this purpose is called power alcohol. It is not sufficiently volatile to give proper starting in cold weather, it is therefore mixed with petrol. A mixture of 25% of power alcohol and 75% petrol has been used in our country as a substitute for petrol. The petroleum resources of India are meagre while alcohol is available in plenty.

Gaseous Fuels

Butane: Gaseous hydrocarbons from petroleum contain propane and butane. They are seperated and compressed in steel cylinders and are used in furnances, internal combustion engines or for cooking.

Methane: It is the main component (90%) of natural gas. In addition being a fuel it is the biggest source for hydrogen. Hydrogen is generally converted to ammonia for the fertilizer industry.

$$CH_4 \xrightarrow[\text{catalyst}]{1400k} C + 2H_2 \qquad \xrightarrow{N_2/\text{catalyst}} NH_3$$

$$CH_4 + H_2O \xrightarrow{1300k} CO + 3H_2 \xrightarrow{N_2/\text{catalyst}} NH_3$$

Water gas

It is obtained by passing steam over red hot coke.

It is a mixture of equal volumes of CO and H_2.

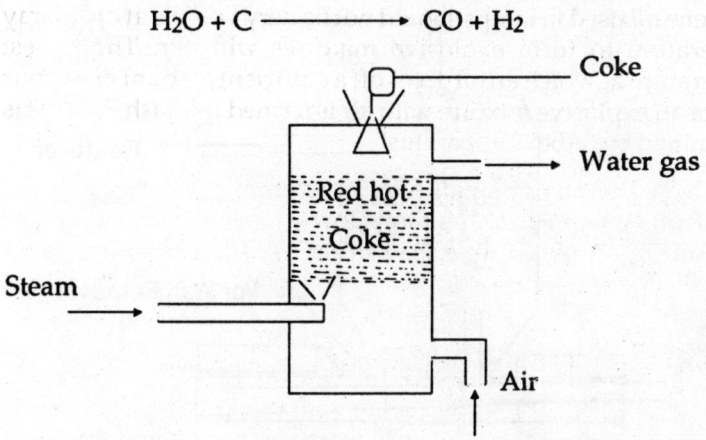

$$H_2O + C \longrightarrow CO + H_2$$

Fig. 9.4 Manufacture of water gas.

The reaction is endothermic. The red hot coke begins to cool down after some time and has to be reheated by passing a hot blast of air. The process is therefore intermittent and consists in passing an alternate blast of air and steam. It burns with non-luminous flame.

Uses of water gas

(i) as a fuel gas.

(ii) as a source of commercial hydrogen.

(iii) as an illuminating gas, when

mixed with C_2H_2 or C_2H_4 which burn with a luminous flame. The gas so formed is called carburetted water gas.

(iv) In the manufacture of methyl alcohol.

Producer Gas

It is prepared by passing air through a tower containing red hot coke. The oxygen of the air combines with carbon to form carbon monoxide.

$$2C + O_2 \longrightarrow 2CO$$

It consists of about one third of its volume of nitrogen (from air). The reaction being exothermic, subsequent heating of the coke is not required.

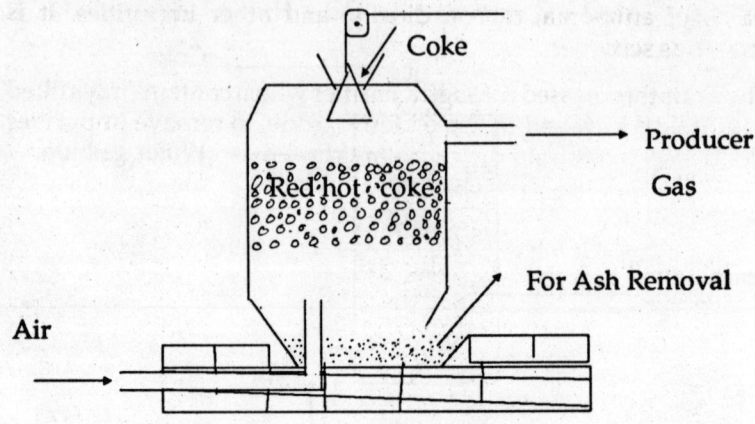

Fig. 9.5. Production of Producer gas.

Producer gas is largely used in metallurgical processes owing to a high temperature produced by its combustion and to its cleanliness and convenience.

Coal Gas

It is prepared by the destructive distillation of coal in fire clay retorts. The plant is shown in Fig. 9.6. The vapours from the retort pass into the hydraulic main where they pass through the water, get cooled and some ammonia is disolved out and a certain amount of coal tar is deposited.

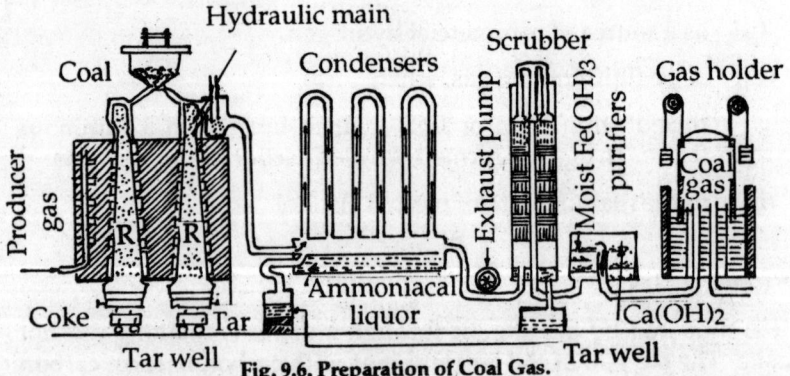

Fig. 9.6. Preparation of Coal Gas.

The retorts, R Rare made of fire clay.

The gas then passes through the condenser which are vertical iron tubes. These tubes cool the gases completely and volatile liquids are condensed in the form of coal tar and ammonical liquors. The gas is then passed through a tower packed with coke from the top of which stream of water falls. It washes the gas and removes the last traces of ammonia, carbon dioxide and other impurities. It is known as scrubber.

The gas is then passed through a purifier which contains trays filled with slaked lime and hydrated ferric oxide, to remove impurities like carbon dioxide, hydrogen sulphide and carbon disulphide.

$$Ca(OH)_2 + CO_2 \longrightarrow CaCO_3 + H_2O$$

$$Ca(OH)_2 + 2H_2S \longrightarrow Ca(HS)_2 + 2H_2O$$

$$Ca(HS)_2 + CS_2 \longrightarrow CaCS_3 + H_2S$$
$$\text{calcium}$$
$$\text{thiocarbonate}$$

$$Fe_2O_3 + 3H_2S \longrightarrow Fe_2S_3 + 3H_2O$$

To remove cyanide, the gas is passed through purifier containing ferrous sulphate and alkali, when ferrocyanide is formed.

$$NaOH + HCN \longrightarrow NaCN + H_2O$$

$$FeSO_4 + 6Na\,CN \longrightarrow Na_4\,Fe(CN)_6 + Na_2SO_4$$

The purified gas is then stored in a gas holder from where it is supplied through pipes to the consumer.

Uses

(i) The main use of a coal gas is as a gaseous fuel and as an illuminant. The luminosity of the coal gas flame is due to the presence of unsaturated hydrocarbons like ethylene and vapours of naphthalene and benzene.

(ii) It is used to provide an inert atmosphere in a number of preprations and

(iii) To provide a reducing atmosphere in metallurgical operations etc.

Marsh Gas

Methane is the principal product of organic decay in swamps and marshes, the gas being set free by the action of bacteria, this method of formation in nature has given rise to the name 'Marsh gas' for methane. Sewage sludge which has been fermented by bacteria yields a gas containing about 70% methane and this is used as a liquid fuel.

Advantages of Gaseous Fuel

The gaseous fuels have the following advantages over solid and liquid fuels.

1. Gaseous fuel burn with a limited supply of air. It is free from ash and other foreign matter.

2. They burn efficiently and high temperature is reached in seconds.

3. They can be fed into the furnance by a pipe. No physical handling of the fuel is required. The temperature of the furnance is easily controlled.

4. They are economical as no extra fuel is required to heat them. There is less loss of heat than solid and liquid fuels.

Combustion

A chemical reaction in which a combustible substance burns in air and is accompanied by evolution of heat and light is called combustion.

Calculation for minimum quantity of air required for the complete combustion of 1kg. of solid or liquid fuel. It can be calculated if the percentage composition of the fuel is known. The elements generally present in a fuel which undergo combustion are C, H, S and O. The oxygen present in air and fuel reacts with C, H and S during combustion of the fuel.

The following are the steps involved in the calculations

(a) Let the weight of C, H, S and O present per kg. of the fuel be C, H, S and O respectively.

(b) With the help of chemical equation, the quantity of air required for complete combustion of C kg. of carbon H kg of hydrogen, S kg of sulphur is given as under:

(i) Combustion of carbon

$$C + O_2 \longrightarrow CO_2$$

12   32

12 kg. of carbon need 32 kg. of oxygen for complete combustion.

$\therefore$ C kg. of carbon will require $\dfrac{32}{12} \times C$ kg of oxygen = 2.67 C kg.

(ii) Combustion of hydrogen

$$2H_2 + O_2 \rightarrow 2H_2O$$

$$\begin{array}{cc} 4 & 32 \\ \text{or } 2 & 16 \end{array}$$

2 kg of hydrogen need sixteen kg of oxygen for complete combustion.

∴ H kg of hydrogen will require $\dfrac{16}{2} \times$ H kg of oxygen = 8 H kg.

(iii) Combustion of sulphur

$$S + O_2 \rightarrow SO_2$$

$$32 \quad 32$$

32 kg of S need 32 kg of oxygen for complete combustion.

∴ S kg of S will require $\dfrac{32}{32} \times$ S kg of oxygen = S kg

Therefore quantity of oxygen required for the combustion of 1 kg of fuel is

$$(2.67 \times C + 8H + S)kg$$

But O kg of oxygen is already present in 1 kg of fuel. Therefore the correct quantity of oxygen required for the combustion of 1 kg of fuel is

$$(2.67 \times C + 8H + S - O) \, kg$$

But air consists of 23% of oxygen by weight, therefore the quantity of air required will be

$$(2.67 \, C + 8H + S - O) \times \frac{100}{23} \, kg.$$

Problems on combustion reactions

Exercise 1. A fuel on analysis have the following results C = 85.8%, H = 12.5%, S = 1.5%, and O = 0.2% Calculate the minimum quantity of air required for complete combustion of 1 kg of fuel. (Air consist of 23% of Oxygen by weight)

Solution: Amount of carbon present in 1 kg of fuel = $\dfrac{85.8}{100}$ = 0.858 kg

Amount of hydrogen = $\dfrac{12.5}{100}$ = 0.125 kg

Amount of sulphur = $\dfrac{1.5}{100}$ = 0.015 kg

$$\text{Amount of oxygen} = \frac{0.2}{100} = 0.002 \text{ kg}$$

Substituting these values in the equation

$$\text{Air required} = (2.67 \text{ c} + 8H + S - O) \times \frac{100}{23} \text{ kg}$$

We get $(2.67 \times 0.858 + 8 \times 0.125 + 0.015 - 0.002) \times \frac{100}{23} \text{ kg} =$ 14.33 kg.

Nuclear - Plutonium, Uranium

Uranium has two isotopes; $_{92}U^{235}$ and $_{92}U^{238}$. $_{92}U^{235}$ occurs only to the extent of 0.7% in natural uranium. When $_{92}U^{235}$ is bombarded with slow moving neutrons (from cosmic rays) the whole

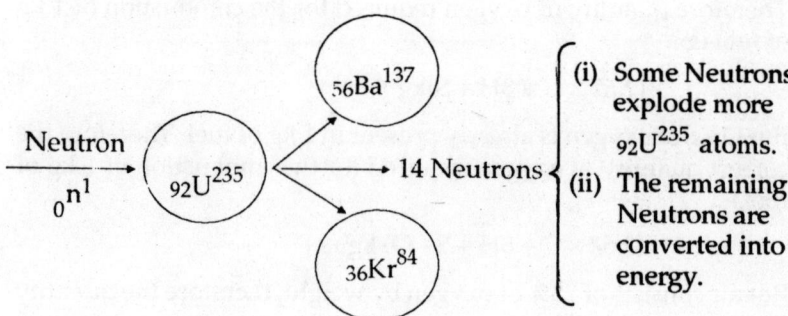

nucleus splits up into two massive nuclei one of barium $_{56}Ba^{137}$ and the other of $_{36}Kr^{84}$ with 14 extra neutrons coming out in the process. This process is known as nuclear fission. Some of these neutrons so librated attack other uranium nuclei and thus cause a chain reaction while others are converted into energy.

In an atom bomb this fission of $_{92}U^{235}$ proceeds uncontrolled and the immense amount of energy set free by the chain reaction is responsible for the havoc that it can cause to life and property. This chain reaction can be controlled in a device known as nuclear reactor, the energy from which can be used for running power plants.

Plutonium which does not occur in nature, can be prepared artifically from $_{92}U^{238}$ (more abundant isotope).

$$_{92}U^{938} + _{0}n^{1} \longrightarrow _{92}U^{239} \longrightarrow _{93}Np^{239} + _{-1}e^{0}$$

uranium   Neptunium B-particle
isotope

The uranium isotope $_{92}U^{239}$ has a short half-life period and is quickly converted into neptunium. This new element 93 has a short half-life period of 2.3 days and after emitting a beta particle is converted to plutonium which is element 94.

$$_{93}Np^{239} \longrightarrow _{94}Pu^{239} + _{-1}e^{0}$$

Plutonium   B-particle

Its half-life period was found to be 24,000 years. Thus it is quite stable. Being chemically distinct from uranium, it can easily be seperated by chemical means. It can also undergo nuclear fission in a manner similar to $_{92}U^{235}$ when bombarded with neutrons. The reactors have been built to produce plutonium fo military purposes and produce electricity.

Many small power plants have been designed and are being planned to propel vessels and vehicles and aircrafts. The sub-marine Nautilus which started its cruise Jan. 1955 was the first of the fleet of nuclear powered under sea craft to be built. Since then many more have been built.

QUESTIONS

1.   (a) What is a fuel? Give the different types of fuel?

   (b) What are the important requirements of fuel to be used in an industry?   (W. 1989)

2.   (a) How is coal analysed? Describe in detail proximate and ultimate analysis.

   (b) Give the composition of the following gaseous fuels:

   1. Natural gas 2. Water gas 3. Producer gas 4. Bio gas 5. Oil gas.   (S-1989)

3.   (a) What are the advantages of gaseous fuel?

   (b) Describe giving a neat sketch the manufacture of water gas

   (c) On analysis, an oil was found to have the following composition.

   C = 84% H = 12% O = 4%

Find the weight of air required for the complete burning of 1 kg of this oil. (Air contains 23% of Oxygen by weight). (W-1988)

4. Calculate the weight and volume of air required for the combustion of 1 kg of carbon.

(C = 12, O = 16, are the atomic weight)

Assume air contains 23% by wt. of Oxygen and 21% by volume of nitrogen. (S-1990)

5. (a) Discuss the advantages and disadvantages of solid, liquid and gaseous fuels over each other.

(b) Write notes on the following:

(i) Preparation of Producer gas. (ii) Bio gas plant.

6. (a) What is a fuel? Give the different types of fuels.

(b) What are the important requirements of fuels to be used in an industry.

(c) Calculate the volume of air containing 20% oxygen by volume at 27°C and 760 mm pressure which will be required for complete combustion of 1 KG of coal containing C = 80% H_2 = 15% and rest incumbustible matter. (W-1989)

7. Give an account of the manufacture of coal gas and name its important constituents.

8. A fuel contains 90% of carbon and 10% of incombustible matter. What volume of air at N.T.P. (containing 21% by volume of Oxygen) will be required to burn completely 1 Kilogram of this fuel.

9. Name the different useful products from petroleum. Give one use of each.

10. How is petroleum produced in nature? Name the leading petroleum producing countries in the world.

11. Say in Yes or No.

(i) Coke is used in the preparation of water gas.

(ii) Kerosene oil is used in sweets.

(iii) Lubricating oil is used as a lubricant.

(iv) Water gas is CO + H_2

12. Select the correct answers.

    (i) The % of carbon in lignite is a) 11% b) 20% c) 70% d) 100 %

    (ii) Producer gas is a mixture of:

    a) CO + N₂ b) C0₂ + N₂ c) CO + H₂ d) CO₂ + H₂

    (iii) Coal gas is obtained by

    (a) the destructive distillation of coal.

    (b) the fractional distillation of coal.

    (c) heating coal with steam.

    (d) heating coal to very high temperature under pressure.

13. *Fill in the blanks:*

    (i) Our laboratory gas is produced from ---------------

    (ii) Fuel used in railway engine is ---------------

    (iii) Fuel used in open hearth furnace is ---------------

    (iv) Water gas is a mixture of ---------------

    (v) Bomb calorimeter is used to determine the calorific value of ---------------.   (S-1988)

ANSWERS

3. c. 13.7 kg. 4.11.593 kg and 2362·8 litrs.

6. 12820·lits 8. 8000 litres at NTP

11. i) Yes ii) No. iii) Yes iv) Yes

12. i) c ii) a iii) a

13. a) Kerosene oil ii) Diesel oil iii) Producers gas iv) CO + H₂ v) Soild and liquid fuels.

Chapter X

Lubricants

Defination: Latin verb 'Lubricare' meaning "to make slippery", is to reduce friction, any substance-liquid, solid or gaseous-capable of controlling friction and wear between surfaces can be classed as a lubricant. In many machines, cooling by the lubricants is equally important. The lubricant may also be called upon to prevent rusting and deposition of solids on close fitting parts. Liquid, plastic and solid material are used as lubricants, although sound design requires the appliction of liquid lubricants where ever possible.

Types of lubrications

The following are three types:

(a) Fluid film lubrication (b) Extreme pressure lubrication and (c). Boundary lubrication.

We will discuss only the first two as per syllabus.

(a) *Fluid film lubrication.*

Interposing a fluid film that completely separates the sliding surfaces results in fluid film lubrication (Fig. 10.1). The fluid may be introduced intentionally, as the oil in the main bearings of an automobile (or un-intentionally as in the case of water between a smooth rubber tire and a wet payment). Although the fluid is usually a liquid such as oil, water and a wide range of other materials, it may also be a gas. The gas most commonly employed is air.

To keep the parts separated, it is necessary that the pressure within the lubricating film balance the load on the sliding surfaces (if the lubricating film's pressure is supplied by an external source, the system is said to be lubricated hydrostatically). If the pressure between the surfaces, is generated as a result of the shape and motion of the surfaces themselves, (however) the system is hydro-dynamically lubricated.

This (second) type of lubrication depends upon the viscious properties of the lubricant. Light machines like watches, clocks, guns, sewing machines, scientific equipments etc are provided with this type of lubrications.

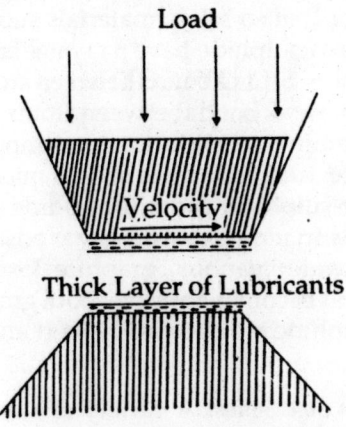

Fig. 10.1. Fluid film lubrication.

(b) Extreme pressure lubrication:

Certain types of gears (particularly the hypoids used in automotive rear-axle transmission) operate under such severe condition of load and sliding speed, with resulting high temperature and pressure that ordinary lubricants cannot provide complete protection against metal contact, this leads to welding, transfer of surface metal, and ultimate destruction of the gears. (Also, in certain machining operations, it is necessary to prevent the chip from welding to the cutting tool). For such applications lubricants containing sulphur and chlorine compounds are used. At the temperature developed in the contact, these react chemically with the metal surfaces, the resulting sulphide and chloride films provide penetration resistant, low-shear strength films which prevent damages to the surfaces. Care in formulating these lubricants must, however, be exercised to ensure that corrosion of metal at normal temperature does not occur.

Classification of lubricants:

Lubricants can be divided into

i) Solid ii) Semi-solid and iii) Liquid

    A.   Solid Lubricants: A solid lubricant is a film of solid material interposed between two rubbing surfaces to reduce friction and wear. The films may consist of inorganic or organic compounds or of metal.

Inorganic compounds: There are three general types of inorganic compounds that serve as solid lubricants:

1. *Layer-lattice or laminar solids:* materials such as graphite and molybdenum disulphide have a crystal lattice structure arranged in layers. Strong bonds between atoms within a layer and relatively weak bonds between atoms of different layers allow the lamina to slide on one another. Other such materials are tungsten disulphide, mica, boron nitride, borax, silver-sulphate, cadmium iodide and lead iodide. Graphites low friction is due largely to adsorbed films, in the absence of water vapour, graphite loses its lubricating properties and becomes abrasive. Both graphite and molybdenum disulphide are chemically inert and have high thermal stability.

2. *Miscellaneous Soft Solids:* A variety of solids such as white lead, lime, talc, bentonite, silver iodide and lead monoxide are used as lubricant.

3. *Chemical Conversion Coatings:* A number of inorganic compounds can be formed on the surface of a metal by chemical reactions. The best known such lubricating coatings are sulphide, chloride, oxide, phosphate and oxalate films.

Solid Organic Compounds: There are two general classes of solid organic lubricants:

1. *Soap, Waxes and fats:* This class includes metallic soaps of aluminium, calcium, sodium, lithium, animal waxes such as bees wax, fatty acids such as stearic and palmitic acids; and fatty esters such as lard and tallow.

2. Polymeric films: These are the synthetic substances such as poly tetra-fluoroethylene and polychlorofluoroethylene. One major advantage of such film-type lubricants is their resistance to deterioration during exposure to the elements. Very thin films of such polymers also serve as protective coatings, as well as lubricants for many types of industrial machinery subjected to great variations in temperature and humidity.

Metal films: Thin films of soft metal on a hard substrate can act as effective lubricants if the adhesion to the substrate is good. Such metals include lead, tin and indium.

B. *Semi-solid lubricants:* A lubricating grease is a semi solid lubricant consisting of a thickening agent in a liquid lubricant. Soaps of aluminium, barium, calcium, lithium, sodium, and strontium are the major thickening agents. Non-soap thickeners consists of such inorganic compounds as modified clays, fine silicas. Solids, usually referred to as fillers, are sometimes added in concentration upto several percent. Fillers are normally inorganic materials such as asbestos, graphite, metal oxides, metal powders, or metal sulphides. Additives are frequently incorporated to resist oxidation and corrosion and to improve film strength.

Lubrication by grease may prove more desirable than lubrication by oil under conditions when (i) less frequent lubricant application is necessary (ii) grease acts as a seal against loss of lubricant and ingress of contaminants (iii) less dripping or splattering of lubricant is called for, or (iv) less sensitivity to inaccuracies in the mating parts is needed.

C. *Liquid lubricants:* Depending on their origin, they are classified as:

1. Animal and vegetable lubricants: Animal and vegetable products were certainly man's first lubricants and were used in large quan-tities. But because they lack chemical inertness and because lubrication requirements have become more demanding, they have been largely superseded by petroleum products and by synthetic materials (Some organic substances such as lard oil and sperm oil are still in use as additive because of their special lubricating properties).

2. Petroleum lubricants:-Petroleum lubricants are predominantly hydrocarbon products extracted from fluids that occur naturally within the earth. They are used widely as lubricants because they posses a combination of the following desirable properties (i) availability in suitable viscosities (ii) low volatility (iii) inertness (resistance to deterioration of the lubricant) (iv) Corrosion protection (resistance to deterioration of the sliding surfaces) and (v) low cost.

With improvement in refining methods, it has been possible to produce high quality lubricants from a variety of crudes. Lubricants are refined from crude petroleum by various processes: (1) Vacuum distillation, (2) Solvent extraction (3) Solvent dewaxing (using solvents to remove wax), (4) hydrofining (treating with hydrogen in the presence of a catalyst).

3. *Synthetic lubricants:* Synthetic lubricants generally can be characterized as oily, neutral liquid materials not usually obtained directly from petroleum but having some properties similar to petroleum lubricants.

Interest in synthetics has increased greatly-more to meet some of the advance demands of technology than because of any critical shortage of petroleum lubricants. Among the improved properties offered by synthetics are low volatility, stability of viscosity with temperature changes, resistance to oxidation and fire resistance. Since the properties of synthetics vary considerably, each synthetic lubricant tends to find a special application. Below are given some synthetic lubricants and their typical application.

Synthetic Lubricant	Typical Uses
Dibasic acid esters	Instrument oil, jet Terbine lubricant, hydraulic fluid.
Phosphate esters	Fire resistant, hydraulic fluid, low temperature lubricant.
Silicate esters	Heat transfer fluid, high temperature hydraulic fluid.
Fluorol compounds	Non-inflammable fluid, extreme oxidation resistant lubricant.

Characteristic of lubricants

The following are the important properties of lubricants:

1. *Viscosity:* The viscosity of a liquid is defined as the ratio of the shearing stress to the rate of shear or is the resistance in a liquid to flow. It determines the amount of friction that will be encountered between sliding surfaces and whether a thick film can be built to avoid wear from solid to solid contact. Viscosity customarily is measured by a viscometer, which determines the flow rate of the lubricant under standard conditions; the higher the flow rate, the lower the viscosity. Lubricants with low viscosity are generally preferred for bearing subjected to high speed and low pressure. Whereas lubricants with high viscosity are recommended for low speed and high pressure.

2. *Viscosity Index:* Since little change of viscosity with fluctuations in temperature is desirable to keep variations in friction at a minimum, fluids frequently are rated in terms of viscosity index. The less the viscosity is changed by temperature higher the viscosity index.

3. *Oiliness:* The term relates to a lubricant's tendency to wet and adhere to a surface under conditions of heavy pressure or load. When a lubricant oil of poor oiliness is subjected to high pressure, it has a tendency to be squeezed out of the lubricated machine parts, thereby its lubricantion action stops. On the other hand, lubricants which have good oiliness stay in between the lubricated surfaces when they are subjected to high pressure.

   Oiliness is a very important property of lubricants, particularly for extreme pressure lubrication. Mineral oils have got very poor oiliness. Animal and vegetable oils and fatty acids are considered to be high in oiliness. So, in order to improve the oiliness of mineral oils additives like vegetable oils and fatty acids (such as oleic and stearic acids) are added to them. (There is no formal test for the measurement of oiliness, determination of this factor is chiefly through subjective judgement and experience.)

4. *Acidity:* Determination of acidic consituents is referred to as "acid number". Which is defined as the number of milligrams of KOH required to neutralize the free acid in 1 gm of the lubricant. Acidity causes the corrosion of the bearing and is harmful. It increases if the lubricant suffers oxidising action during lubricating action. A lubricating oil should possess acid value less than 0.1 . Any value greater than 0.1 indicates the oil has oxidised.

Determination of Acidity:

A known weight (about 5-10 gm) of the oil and 50 ml of alcohol are taken in a flask. The flask is then heated over a water bath for about $\frac{1}{2}$ hour. The contents of the flask are then titrated against N/10 KOH using phenolphthalein as indicator. Then acid value is calculated as under:

$$\text{Acid value} = \frac{\text{No. of ml of } N/10 \text{ KOH used} \times 5.6}{\text{Weight of oil taken in gram}}$$

Where 5.6 is the amount of KOH present in 1 ml of N/10 KOH.

5. *Emulsification:* It is the property of oils to get intimataely mixed with water forming a mixture called emulsion. Certain oils from emulsion with water easily. Emulsions have a tendency to pick up dirt, grit, foreign matter etc. thereby causing abrasion and wearing out of the lubricated parts of the machinery. So a good lubricating oil should not form any

emulsion and if it forms, then the emulsion should break off quickly.

6. *Flash Point:* It is the lowest temperature at which the oil lubricant gives off enough vapours so as to form an explosive mixture that will flash, if brought into contact with flame. Flash point may in some instances become the major consideration in selecting the proper lubricant, especially in lubricating machinery handling highly flammable material. A good lubricant should have flash point at least above the temperature at which it is to be used.

7. *Fire Point:* It is the lowest temperature at which the vapours of the oil burns continuously for at least five seconds, when a tiny flame is brought near it. In most case the fire points are 5 to $40°$ higher than the flash points. The flash and fire point are important when oil is exposed to high temperature service.

8. *Volatility:* It is the tendency of the lubricant to evaporate. Working with lubricating oils in heavy machinery at high temperature, a portion of oil may vaporize leaving behind a residual oil which have different lubricating properties like increase viscosity. A good lubricant should have low volatility.

9. *Pour point:* It is a temperature at which lubricant ceases to flow, is of importance in appraising flow properties at low temperature. As such it can become the determining factor in selecting the one lubricant from among a group with identical properties.

10. *Saponification Value:* It is given by the number of milligrams of KOH required to saponify 1 gm of oil. Mineral oils do not safonify at all, but vegetable and animal oils do. This test helps to find whether the oil under reference is animal and vegetable oil or mineral oil or a compounded oil containing vegetable and mineral oils.

Determination of Saponification value:

A known weight (about 5 gm) of the oil and 50 ml of N/2 KOH solution in alcohol are taken in a flask. The flask is heated over a water- bath for about an hour, using a reflux condenser. The unreacted KOH in the flask is then back titrated against N/2 HCl using phenolphthalein as indicator. Then saponification value is calculated as under:

Saponification Value = No. of ml of - N/2 KOH taken –

$$\frac{\text{No. of ml of N/2 acid used for back titrations}}{\text{Wt. of oil in g taken for saponification}} \times 28$$

Every oil as got a definite saponification value and if it is less or more than this, it is probably adulterated.

Selection of lubricants for different types of machinery

Every lubricant application is specially formulated to meet its unique requirements. For example, if a lubricant used at high temperature undergo volatalization of a portion of it leaving behind a residual oil which has different lubricating properties like higher viscosity. Such a lubricant should not be used. A few applications in which special charcteristics are desirable and lubricant recommanded are given in the table below:

Typical special purpose lubricants

Lubricant application	Lubricant properties of special interest	Lubricant recommended.
1. Steam turbine	High oxidation resistance corrosion resistance, good water seperation, low foaming.	Lubricating oils compounded with suitable additives.
2. Transformers	High dielectric strength, low viscosity, oxidation resistance, highly resistivity.	Highly refined mineral oils properly filtered and dried.
3. Gears	High film strength, oxidation resistance, corrosion resistance.	Mineral lubricating oils containing extreme pressure additive (like metallic soap & chlorine, sulphur or phosphrous).
4. Internal combustion engines	High viscosity index, high thermal stability.	Petroleum oils containing additives.
5. Steam engine cylinders	High viscosity, high metal weting, least tendency to gumming at high temperature	Steam refined paraffin base, mineral oil compounded with fixed oil (vegetable and animal oils)
6. Delicate instruments (watches, clocks, sewing machines scientific instruments)	Not exposed to high temperature extreme load or water	Thin vegetable & animal oils like palm.
7. Cutting tools	Low viscosity, cooling, prevent rust and corrosion, fine finish	(a) Heavy cuttings, mineral oils of low viscosity with additives like fatty oil and chlorinated compounds (b) Light cuttings oil emulsion

QUESTIONS

1.   a. Classify the common lubricants and discuss their properties and uses.

       b. Define the following term as applied to lubricants:

       i) Fire and flash point

       ii) Volatility

       iii) Saponification value

       iv) Emulsification

       v) Viscosity index.

       c. Choose and rewrite the correct answer:

       i) Good lubricant should have low/high viscosity index

       ii) Under extremely high temperature solid/semisolid/liquid lubricants can be used.

       iii) Flash point is higher/lower than fire point

       iv) The oiliness of mineral oil is more/less than vegetable oils

       v) Acid value of vegetable oil is more/less than mineral oils.   (W - 1988)

2.   a. How are lubricants classified? **Give examples.**

       b. Describe the more important physical and chemical methods of testing a lubricant.

       c. Write note on "Selection of proper lubricants" for various equipments/machines etc.   (S - 1989)

3.   a. What are lubricants?

       b. Mention six qualities which are tested for selecting a good lubricant.

       c. Describe methods to estimate any two of the qualities for a good lubricant in detail   (W - 1989)

4.   Write notes on "saponification value of an oil sample".   (S - 1990)

5.   a. Classify the common lubricants and discuss their properties and uses.

       b. Define the following terms as applied to lubricants:

    i) Fire and flash point

    ii) Saponification value

    iii) Emulsification

    c. Write a note on "Selection of a lubricant".   (S - 1988)

ANSWERS

1. c

    i) high viscosity index.

    ii) solid

    iii) lower than fire point.

    iv) less than vegetable oils

    v) more.

Chapter XI

Ores and Minerals

Mineral: Solid compounds of metals occuring in nature are termed minerals. thus NaCl, KCl, $CaCO_3$, ZnS which occur in nature are all minerals.

Ores: Such minerals which are used for commercial preparation of a metal are called its ore. Bauxite Al_2O_3. $2H_2O$ is an ore of aluminium. Zinc blende ZnS is an ore of Zinc.

Ganque: The minerals are invariably contaminated with rock and earthy impurities termed gangue.

Minerals dressing: The process of removal of gangue or matrix from the ore is techanically known as concentration or ore - dressing.

General principles of concentration of ores.

1.   *Froth Floatation Process:* This process is used to concentrate sulphide ores. In this method, the finely powdered-ore is mixed with water and pine oil in a tank. The air is blown through the mixture. A forth is formed. The ore ore particles rise to the surface carried by the froth. The earthy impurities are wetted by water and sink to the bottom as shown in Fig. 11.1

Foam of Sulphide Ore   Air

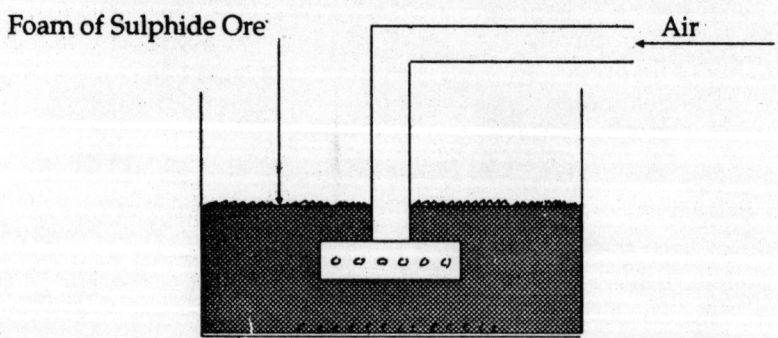

Fig. 11.1. Froth Floatation Process.

The forth is skimmed off. Acid is added to break up the forth. The concentrated ore is filtered and dried.

2. *Magnetic Separation:* This method is used when the ore or the impurity is magnetic in nature. For example tin stone which contains Wolfram (tungstates of iron and manganese $FeWo_4$ & $MnWO_4$) as magnetic impurity is concentrated by this method.

    The powdered ore is dropped over a belt (Fig. 11.2) which is moving over two rollers, one of which is magnetic. Non-magnetic impurities fall down in a separate heap.

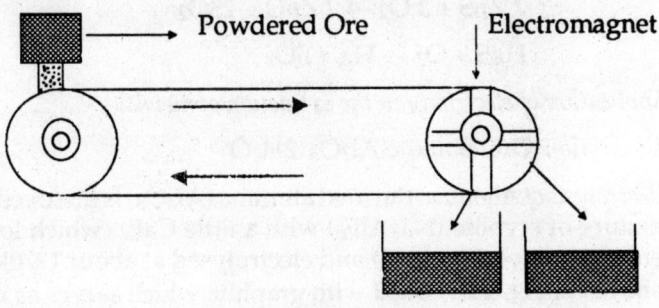

Powdered Ore   Electromagnet

Magnetic Particles   Non Magnetic
                                        Particles

Fig. 11.2. Magnetic Separation.

3. *Washing:* By washing the powdered ore in a current of water, the lighter rocky and earthy impurities can be washed away over much longer distances. The heavier ore particles are left behind.

    Calcination: is the process of heating an ore strongly so that volatile impurities are removed and the decomposable oxy-salts are converted to oxides. Here presence of air is not essential nor it necessary to exclude it. Some examples are:

    $$CaCO_3 \rightarrow CaO + CO_2$$

    $$Al_2O_3 . 2H_2O \rightarrow Al_2O_3 + 2H_2O$$
    $$2Al(OH)_3 \rightarrow Al_2O_3 + 3H_2O$$
    $$CUCO_3 . CU(OH)_2 \rightarrow 2CUO + H_2O + CO_2$$
    $$CaCO_3 . MgCO_3 \rightarrow CaO + MgO + 2CO_2$$

    Roasting: is the process of heating an ore in a controlled supply of air at a regulated temperature so that sulphur, arsenic and other elements present in a free or combined state are oxidised to volatile oxides and the metal oxide is left behind. Sometimes oxidation of sulphides is carried out only to sulphate stage as in the case of lead. Some of the oxidation reactions of sulphide ores are given below:

$$4\ FeS_2 + 11\ O_2 \rightarrow 2Fe_2O_3 + 8\ SO_2$$

$$2\ CU_2S + 3\ O_2 \rightarrow 2CU_2O + 2\ SO_2$$

$$2\ PbS + 3\ O_2 \rightarrow 2\ PbO + 2SO_2$$

$$PbS + 2\ O_2 \rightarrow PbSO_4$$

$$2\ ZnS + 3\ O_2 \rightarrow 2\ ZnO + 2SO_2$$

$$HgS + O_2 \rightarrow Hg + SO_2$$

Application of electricity in the extraction of metals:

Aluminium: Ore: Bauxite $Al_2O_3 . 2H_2O$

Electrolysis of Alumina: Purified alumina (Al_2O_3) is dissoved in fused mixture of cryolite (Na_3AlF_6) with a little CaF_2 (which lowers the temperature of the metal) and electrolysed at about 1270k in a cell (shown in Fig. 11.3) lined with graphite which serves as cathode. The anode consists of a number of graphite rods suspended vertically inside the tank about 5-7 cm above the bottom.

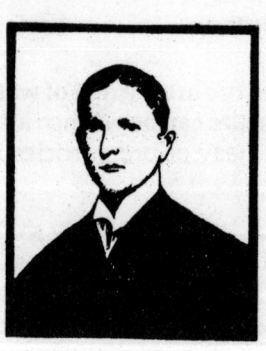

When the current is passed, aluminium is set free at the cathode and collects in the molten state on the floor of the cell while oxygen gas is liberated at the anode. The probable reaction mechanism is as follows:

Charles Martin Hall (1893-1914)

An American Chemist who perfected the electrolytic method for the extraction of Aluminium.

At the cathode $Al^{3+} + 3e^- \rightarrow Al\ (l)$

At the anode $20^{2-} \rightarrow O_2(g) + 4e$

$$C(s) + O_2(g) \rightarrow CO_2(g)$$

The anodic oxygen reacts with carbon anodes giving CO and CO_2. This results in the consumption of the anodes which have to be replaced periodically.

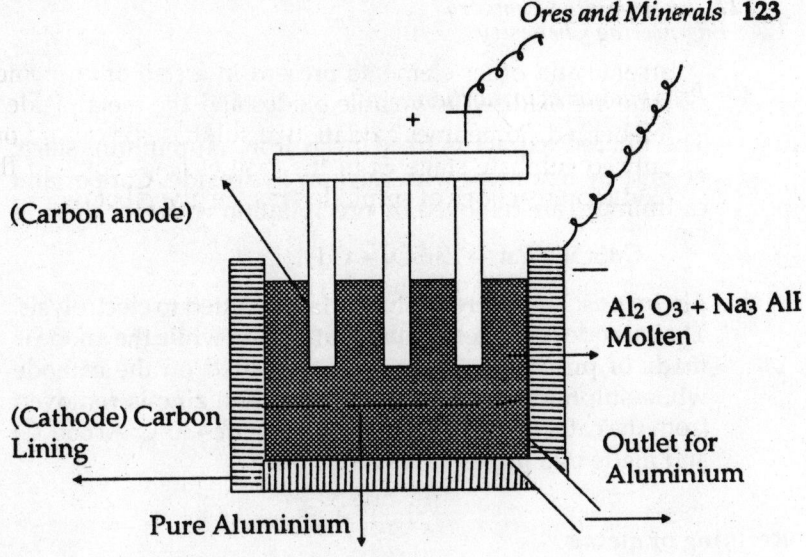

(Carbon anode)

Al₂ O₃ + Na₃ AlF
Molten

(Cathode) Carbon
Lining

Outlet for
Aluminium

Pure Aluminium

Fig. 11.3

Aluminium obtained is 99.5% pure.

Zinc: Ores: Zinc Blende --------- ZnS

Calamine --------- Zn CO₃

Zincite --------- ZnO

Electrolytic Process for the extraction of zinc where electricity is cheap. It involves the following steps:-

1. *Concentration:* If the ore contains iron oxide as impurity the latter is seperated magnetically. Otherwise the siliceous impurities are removed by gravity seperation followed by froth flotation process.

2. *Roasting:* The sulphide ore is roasted to about 700°C carefully when a mixture of zinc oxide and zinc sulphate is formed.

$$ZnS + 2O_2 \rightarrow ZnSO_4$$

$$2ZnS + 3O_2 \rightarrow 2ZnO + 2SO_2$$

3. *Leaching with sulphuric acid:* The roasted ore is extracted with dilute sulphuric acid as also with spent electrolyte from operation (5) Zinc goes in solution as zinc sulphate. Other **soluble sulphates also come in solution.** .

$$ZnO + H_2SO_4 \rightarrow ZnSO_4 + H_2O$$

4. *Precipitation of impurities:*

    The filtered extract is freed from iron, aluminium, silica, arsenic by treatment with calcium hydroxide. Copper and cadmimum are removed by precipitation with zinc dust.

    $$CdSO_4 + Zn \rightarrow ZnSO_4 + Cd$$

5. *Electrolysis:* The filtered solution is submitted to electrolysis. The cathode is a sheet of pure aluminium while the anode is made of pure lead. The zinc is deposited on the cathode while sulphuric acid is regenerated. The zinc is removed from the cathode by melting (m. pt. of zinc $420^{\circ}C$; Al $660^{\circ}C$) and made into ingots. It is 99.95% pure.

Refining of metals

The following are the three methods of refining metals.

1. *Cupellation:* This is employed to purify silver containing lead as an impurity. The impure silver is heated in a shallow vessel made of bone-ash under a blast of air. The lead is easily oxidised to powdery lead monoxide. Most of it is carried away by the blast of air. The rest melts and is absorbed by the bone ash cupel. Pure silver is left behind. Silver itself is not oxidised under these conditions.

2. *Liquation:* is used for refining metals of low melting points. Crude tin may contain some insoluble and non-metallic impurities. By heating such tin (m.p = 505k) on the sloping floor of a furnance purer tin flows down, leaving the impurities behind.

3. *Application of electricity in the refining of metals:*

    Aluminium: *Electrolytic refining:* (Hoope's Process)

    In an iron box lined with carbon at its bottom are three layers of fused mass differing in specific gravity. The upper layer consists of pure aluminium and serves as the cathode. The middle layer consists of a mixture of flourides of Al, Na and Ba. The base layer consists of impure aluminium and acts as the anode. The arrangement of the cell is shown in Fig. 11.4

    On passing the current, aluminium is discharged in the top layer and the middle layer gets an equivalent amount from the base layer. Thus there is gradual transference of Aluminium from base to the top and the impurities are left behind.

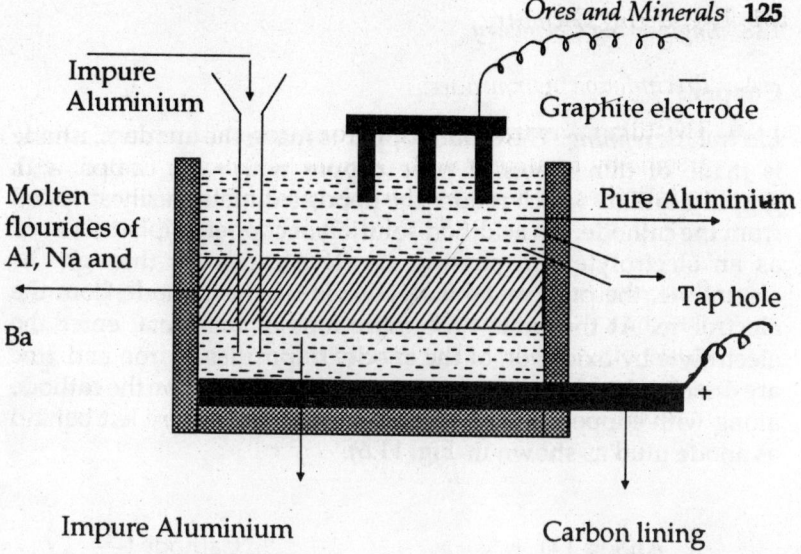

Fig. 11.4. Electrolytic refining of Aluminium.

Aluminium obtained is 99.9% pure.

Zinc

Electrolytic refining: Zinc is purified by electrolytic method using zinc sulphate as an electrolyte, pure zinc wire as the cathode and impure zinc as the anode. On passing current, pure zinc settles at the cathode and the impurities are left at the anode as anode mud. Fig. 11.5

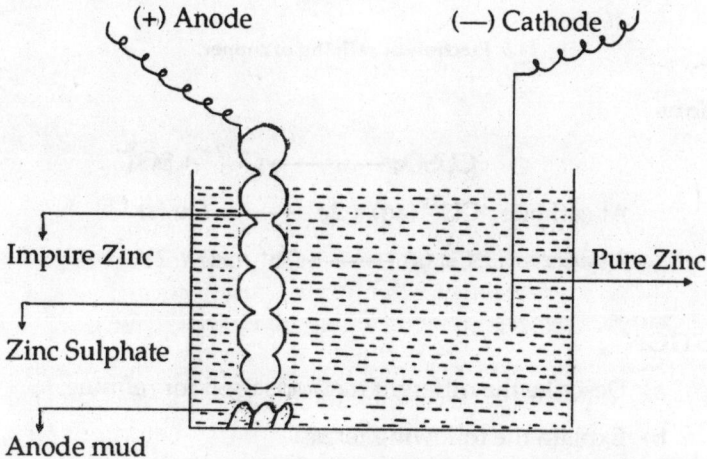

Fig. 11.5. Electrolytic refining of zinc.

Copper

Electrolytic refining: The crude copper is made the anode. Cathode is made of thin sheets of pure copper which are coated with graphite and oil which render the deposited metal easily stripped from the cathode. An acidified solution of copper sulphate is used as an electrolyte. On passing an electric current through the electrolyte, the pure metal is deposited on the cathode from the electrolyte. At the same time more ions of the metal enter the electrolyte by oxidation of the anode. Impurities of iron and zinc are dissolved in electrolyte (which are not deposited on the cathode along with copper) and gold, platinum and silver are left behind as anode mud as shown in **Fig. 11.6).**

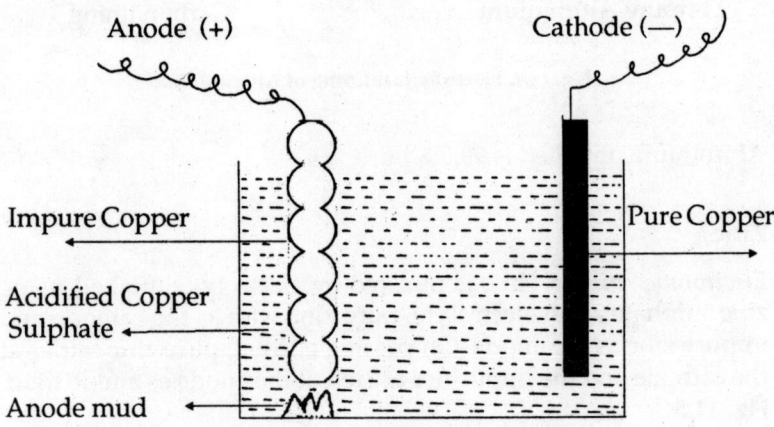

Anode (+)   Cathode (—)

Impure Copper   Pure Copper

Acidified Copper
Sulphate

Anode mud

Fig. 11.6. Electrolytic refining of copper.

Reactions

$$CUSO_4 \longrightarrow CU^{2+} + SO_4^{2-}$$

At cathode : $CU^{2+}(aq) + 2e^- \longrightarrow Cu\ (s)$

At anode   : $Cu\ (s) \longrightarrow Cu^{2+}(aq) + 2e^-$

QUESTION

1.   a) Describe the different methods used for refining.

     b) Explain the following terms:

i) Flux ii) Smelting iii) Cupellation iv) Slag v) Gangue.
(W-1988)

2.   a) Describe briefly the principal steps employed for the extraction of metals from their ores.

Illustrate each step by example.

b) Differentiate the following with suitable examples:

i) Roasting and Calcination.

ii) Flux and Slag iii) Ore and Minerals.

c) Write notes on the following:

i) Types of Metallurgy

ii) electrolytic refining.   (S-1989)

3.   a) Explain the following terms:

i) Flux ii) Slag iii) Gangue.

b) Describe the following.

i) Roasting ii) Smelting

c) Write note on Electro refining.   (W-1989)

4.   a) What is the difference between a mineral and Ore.

b) Explain the following terms (any three)

1) Flux 2) Smelting3) Cupellation 4) Froth-floation process 5) Electro refining.   (S-1990)

5.   a) Describe the different methods used for refining.

b) Outline the methods used for extraction of metals.

c) Complete the following:

i) The process of removing earthy impurties from the ore is known as -----------.

ii) Clay is lighter than the --------------.

iii) In the froth floatation process the powdered ore is agitated with a mixture of ----------.

iv) Oxide ores are generally concentrated by --------------.

v) Flux is a substance used to remove fusibile impurties in the form of --------------.   (S-1988)

6. Complete the following statements.

    i) Sulpide ores are usually concentrated ---------

    ii) Copper is concentrated by --------------.

    iii) Heating of ore in the presence of air is called ------.

    iv) Carbonate ores are usually subjected to ---------.

    v) Smelting is usually done -----------furnace.   (S-1990)

7. Choose and rewrite th correct answer to the following:

    i) Sulphide Ores are generally concentrated by:

      a) Gravity separation process b) Froth floatation process.

    ii) Carbonate ores are generally subjected to

      a) Roasting b) Calcination.

    iii) Heating of the ore in the free supply of air is termed as

      a) Roasting b) Calcination.

    iv) Smelting is generally carried out in

      a) Reverbratory furnace. b) Blast furnace

    v) Oxides ores are generally concentrated by

      a) Gravity separation process.

      b) Froth floatation process.   (W-1988)

ANSWERS

5.   c). i) Concentration. ii) Ore iii) Pine Oil and water. iv) Washing. v) Slag

6.   i) Froth floatation process.

      ii) -do- in the case of sulphide ore.

      iii) Calcination.

      iv) Calcination

      v) In a blast furnace.

7.   i) b ii) b iii) b iv) b v) a

Chapter XII

Metallurgy of Iron and Steel

Iron Ores and minerals: The following are the chief iron ores:

(1) Haematite	—	Fe_2O_3
(2) Magnetite	—	Fe_3O_4
(3) limonite	—	$2Fe_2O_3.3H_2O$
(4) Siderite	—	$FeCO_3$ which is found mixed with varying proportions of clayey materials.
(5) Iron Pyrites	—	FeS_2, which occur abundantly but are used more as a source of sulphur dioxide for the manufacture of sulphuric acid than a source of iron.

Chemistry of smelting

From metal oxides, metals are obtained by a process known as smelting. This involves two main operations: reduction and removal of impurities as slag. Slag is easily fusible material formed by the combination of basic and acidic oxides. Reduction and slagging operation usually take place together. The substance added for formation of slag is flux. If the impurities are acidic oxides like SiO_2, P_2O_5 lime is added as basic flux.

$$SiO_2 + CaO \text{------------------} CaSiO_3$$

$$P_2O_5 + 3CaO \text{------------------} Ca_3(PO_4)_2$$

For basic impurities like MnO, silica acts as acidic flux.

$$MnO + SiO_2 \text{------------------} MnSiO_3$$

Reduction of oxides

Chemical reduction: A variety of reducing agents are used:

Carbon as charcoal, coal and coke, CO, H_2, metals like Na, Al, Mg, etc are some of the common reducing agent. In case of certain sulphides the partly roasted ore is reduced to the metal by using uncharged sulphide itself as the reducing agent.

When carbon is used as the reducing agent, it is converted to CO.

Examples of a few metals obtained by chemical reduction are given below:

i) $SnO_2 + 2C \rightarrow Sn + 2CO$
   Coke
ii) $2ZnO + 2C \rightarrow 2Zn + 2CO$
   Powdered Coal
iii) $Fe_2O_3 + 3CO \rightarrow 2Fe + 3CO_2$
   Coke
iv) $Cr_2O_3 + 2Al \rightarrow 2Cr + Al_2O_3$
v) $TiCl_4 + 2Mg \rightarrow Ti + 2MgCl_2$
vi) $2Cu_2O + Cu_2S \rightarrow 6Cu + SO_2$

Acidic and Basic fluxes

The substance added for formation of slag is called flux. Slag is easily fusible material formed by the combination of basic and acidic oxides.

Acidic fluxes

For basic impurities like MnO, silica acts as acidic flux.

$$MnO + SiO_2 \rightarrow MnSiO_3$$

Basic fluxes

If the impurities are acidic oxides like SiO_2, P_2O_5, lime is added as basic flux.

$$SiO_2 + CaO \rightarrow CaSiO_3$$

$$P_2O_5 + 3CaO \rightarrow Ca_3(PO_4)_2$$

Manufacture of pig-iron in blast furnace:

Oxide and carbonate ores are generally employed and it involves the following steps;

(i) *Washing:* Clay, sand, and other adhering impurities are removed from the heavy ore by washing with water and the ore is thus concentrated.

(ii) *Calcination:* The concentrated ore is then heated in calcining kilns with free excess of air. As a result of this treatment most of moisture, CO_2, sulphur and arsenic are expelled and ferrous oxide is changed to ferric oxide which is porous less fusible and the desired form of the iron oxide. Hematite and magnetite do not usually need calcination. The powdered ore is sintered to convert it into porous lumps.

(iii) *Smelting:* The calcined ore is then smelted i.e. reduced with carbon in the presence of a flux. This is done in a blast furnace (Fig. 12.1). It is a steel structure lined with fire bricks. 100 ft. high and 25 ft. in diameter at the widest part, narrowing some what towards the top and the bottom to provide a proper flow of the material.

The furnance at the base is provided with (i) small pipes called tuyerers through which hot air is admitted (ii) a tap hole through which molten iron can be drawn (iii) a slag hole for the discharge of the slag. The hot gases leaving at the top are utilized for pre-heating the air blast admitted through tuyerers. The charge consisting of the calcined ore mixed with coke and limestone in the approximate ratio of 4 : 2 : 1 is introduced at the top of the furnance by means of the cup and cone arrangement.

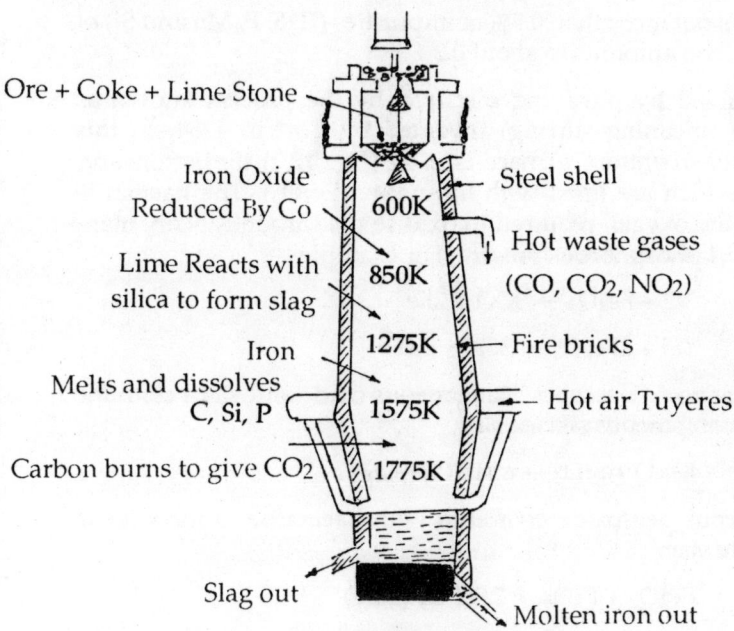

Fig. 12.7. **Blast Furnace.**

Blast of hot air is sent upwards through the tuyerers. A series of reactions take place inside the furnance.

$$CaCO_3 \rightarrow CaO + CO_2$$

$$CO_2 + C \rightarrow 2CO$$

$$2C + O_2 \rightarrow 2CO$$

$$Fe_2O_3 + 3CO \rightarrow 2Fe + 3CO_2$$

$$CaO + SiO_2 \rightarrow CaSiO_3 \text{ (Slag)}$$

Molten iron forms a layer below the slag layer of calcium silicate During melting, iron dissolves some carbon. The slag is removed from the upper hole on the side of the furnance and molten iron is run periodically out from a lower hole into sand moulds to give pig iron.

Cast Iron: Iron obtained from the blast furnance contains about 5% carbon. It is called pig iron. It is also called cast iron as it gives good casting. Cast iron expands slightly on cooling. Cast iron is resistant to corrosion and is used for sewage pipes, lamp posts etc. However it is brittle and very weak for structural uses. A large quantity of cast iron is used in making wrought iron.

Wrought Iron

It contains not more than 0.5% of impurities (C, S, P, Mn and Si) of which carbon amounts to about 0.2%.

It is obtained by purifying cast iron by the process known as puddling (meaning stirring) invented by Cort in 1784. In this process reverberatory furnace is used (Fig. 12.2) the bottom and sides of which are lined with haematite (Fe_2O_3). The haematite supplies the oxygen required to oxidise the carbon, silicon, manganese and phosphorous present. For example

$$3C + Fe_2O_3 \rightarrow 3CO + 2Fe$$

$$3Si + 2Fe_2O_3 \rightarrow 3SiO_2 + 4Fe$$

Carbon monoxide escapes Manganeous oxide and silica combine to form manganeous silicate slag.

$$MnO + SiO_2 \rightarrow MnSiO_3 \text{ (Slag)}$$

Phosphorous pentoxide combines with haematite to form ferric phosphate slag.

$$Fe_2O_3 + P_2O_5 \rightarrow 2FePO_4 \text{ (Slag)}$$

The melting point of iron rises with loss of impurities. Iron, therefore attains a semi-solid state. At this stage it is taken out in the form of balls and the slag squeezed out by hammering. It is then rolled into bars, beaten into sheets or drawn into wires.

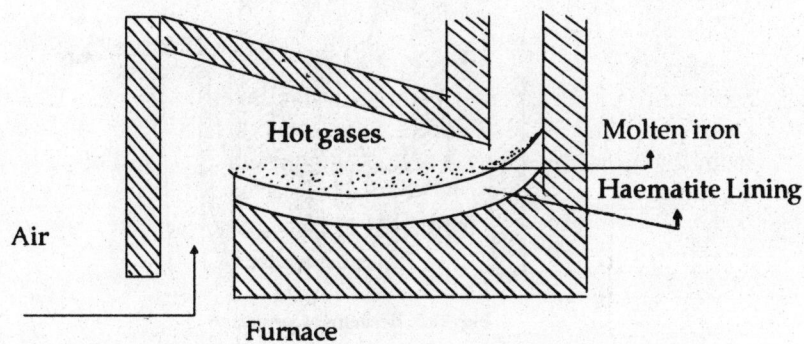

Fig. 12.2. Wrought Iron in Reverberatory furnace.

Properties and uses

Wrought iron contains about 0.2% of carbon besides traces of phosphorous, silicon etc. in the form of slag. It is soft, ductile and malleable and can be welded. Slag gives strength and toughness to the metal and makes it resistant towards rusting and corrosion. It is used in making cores of electromagnets, chains, wire anchors, bolt, nails etc.

Steel

It contains about 0.15% to 1.5% carbon, other elements such as chromium, silicon, nickel, tungsten, vanadium and molybedenum are added for making steel. Number of methods are used in its manufacture. Two important processes are given below:

1. *Bessemer Process:* (1856)

Molten pig-iron from the blast furnance is introduced into Bessemer converter. It is a pear shaped furnance about 20 feet high and 10 feet in diameter. It is made of steel plates and is lined inside with refractory silica bricks. The converter is supported on a central axis. The charging is done while it is in the horizontal position. It is then gradually raised to the vertical position and a blast of hot air is forced into it through the pipes leading to the perforatted bottom of the converters (Fig. 12.3), As the air passes upwards

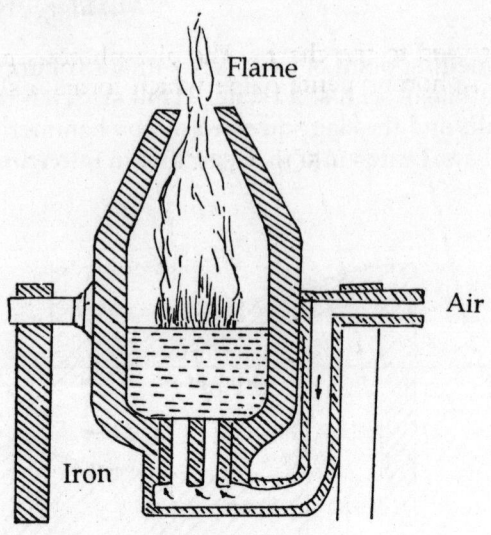

Fig. 12.3. Bessemer Converter.

through the molten metal, it oxidises the impurities (Mn, Si, C) present in pig iron.

$$2Mn + O_2 \rightarrow 2MnO$$

$$Si + O_2 \rightarrow SiO_2$$

$$2C + O_2 \rightarrow 2CO$$

The first effect of the air is to oxidise Mn and Si which passes into the slag as $MnSiO_3$.

$$MnO + SiO_2 \rightarrow MnSiO_3$$

Later on carbon is oxidised to carbon monoxide which burns with a blue flame at the mouth of the converter. When the flame dies out, it indicates that all the carbon has been oxidised. The addition of spiegeleisen (German-mirror iron) (an alloy of Fe, C and Mn) to the molten mass thus prepared adjusts the carbon content and produces manganese steel of the desired quality. It is distributed throughout the mass by blowing in air for some time. To remove blow holes in the product due to bubbles of O_2, N_2 or CO little aluminium or ferrosilicon is also added.

At the end the converter is tilted to pour out the molten steel.

If the pig-iron contains much of phosphorous the converter is lined with lime (CaO) and magnesia (MgO) instead of silica. Some lime is added to the charge. The phosphorous present is oxidised to phosphorous penta oxide which forms a slag of calcium phosphate.

$$4P + 5O_2 \rightarrow 2P_2O_5$$

$$3CaO + P_2O_5 \rightarrow Ca_3 (PO_4)_2 \text{ (Slag)}$$

The slag is known as Thomas slag and is generally used as fertilizer.

2. *Open Hearth Process*: (Siemens and Marten 1910 in England)

The best quality steel is manufactured by this process. The essential principles of this process are:

(i) Oxidation of the impurities present in cast iron by the addition of iron ore instead of passing in air.

(ii) Dilution of the carbon and silicon by the addition of scrap steel or low grade wrought iron.

(iii) The furnance is heated by producer gas working on regenerative system of heat economy.

The charge usually consists of 70-80% of cast iron and 20-30% of scrap iron and haematite. It is melted in an open hearth furnance (40' x 1' x 2') lined with lime or magnesia bricks in the basic process and silica in the acid process Fig. 12.4.

Heating is continued for 8-10 hours. During this time, the impurities get oxidised by haematite.

$$3C + Fe_2O_3 \rightarrow 3CO + 2Fe$$

$$3S + 2Fe_2O_3 \rightarrow 3SO_2 + 4Fe$$

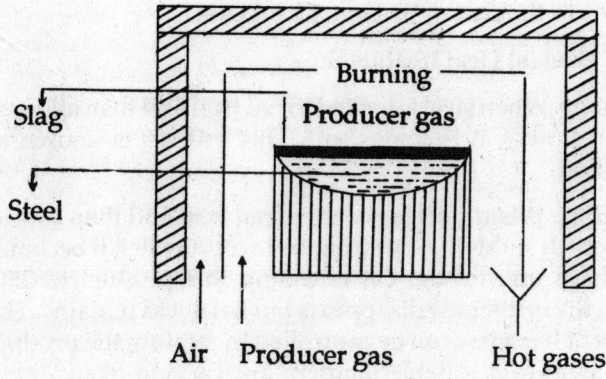

Fig 12.4. The Open Hearth Furnance.

$$3Si + 2Fe_2O_3 \rightarrow 3SiO_2 + 4Fe$$

$$6P + 5Fe_2O_3 \rightarrow 3P_2O_5 + 10Fe$$

Carbon is removed as CO while sulphur escapes as SO_2. Si and P are also oxidised and converted into their respective slags.

$$SiO_2 + CaO \rightarrow CaSiO_3$$

$$P_2O_5 + 3CaO \rightarrow Ca_3(PO_4)_2$$

Samples are drawn out from time to time and examined for carbon content. The requiste amount of spiegeleisen (an alloy of iron, manganese and carbon) and ferro silicon (to remove bubbles due to O_2, N_2 or CO) along with other metals if desired are added at the appropriate stage to get high grade steel with the required composition.

This process has the following advantages:

i) Steel of better quality is obtained.

ii) Scrap iron and iron ore are directly changed into steel.

iii) The process works on regenerative system of heat economy.

iv) The composition of the product and the temperature can be easily controlled.

v) No iron is wasted as slag.

Disadvantages

1. In the case of open hearth process, it takes 8-10 hours to complete whereas Bessemer's process takes 10-20 minutes.

2. Open hearth process needs high capital investment whereas it is low in the case of Bessemer's process.

Properties of steel (a) Heat treatment:

1. *Annealing:* When steel is heated to red heat and then allowed to cool slowly, it becomes soft. This process is known as annealing.

2. *Tempering:* When steel is heated to red heat and then cooled (quenched) suddenly, by plunging in oil or water, it becomes very hard and brittle. On reheating this product to 250-300°C, the brittleness disappears but hardness remains. The degree of hardness can be controlled by heating the product once again to a suitable temperature varying from 200 to 350°C (depending upon the hardness required) then allow-

ing it to cool slowly. This process is known as tempering and is employed for bringing the steel into a suitable state of hardness and elasticity. The temperature to which steel is heated is judged from the colour of the thin oxide film formed on the surface and varies from pale yellow 230°C, to brown 260°C to blue 300°C as the temperature rises. Steel for cutting blades and tools is made yellow but that required for springs, saws, etc. is tempered blue.

3. *Nitriding:* It is employed for surface hardening of steel. It is carried out by heating steel containing 1% aluminium in a current of ammonia at 500-600°C where in nitrogen of ammonia reacts with iron and aluminium surface forming iron and aluminium nitrides giving very strong and durable surface.

   (b) *Alloy steels:* The addition of small quantities of other metals like Mn, Cr, W, Ni, Mo to steel modify its properties, we get an alloy steel, Most important example of alloy steel is the stainless steel (Chief components Cr-18%, Ni-8% and rest steel). It does not rust or corrode and is used for making household utensils, shaving blades, watch-cases etc.

Properties of Iron

Physical:

Pure iron is greyish in colour has melting point 1525°C, boiling point 2450°C and specific gravity 7.85. It is highly magnetic and loses this property above 766°C. It is good conductor of heat and electricity.

Chemical : i) Action of air: In the presence of moist air and carbon dioxide, iron gets covered with a layer of rust consisting of ferric hydroxide and ferric oxide.

On heating in air forms ferroso ferric oxide.

$$3Fe + 2O_2 \text{-------------------} Fe_3O_4$$

ii) With water: Iron decomposes steam.

$$3Fe + 4H_2O \text{------------------} Fe_3O_4 + 4H_2$$

iii) With dil HNO_3: It gives NH_4NO_3.

$$4\,Fe + 10\,HNO_3 \text{--------------} 4\,Fe\,(NO_3)_2 + NH_4NO_3 + 3\,H_2\,O$$

With conc. HNO₃:

Fairly strong nitric acid gives ferric nitrate and a miture of the oxides of nitrogen.

$$Fe + 6 HNO_3 \text{----------------} Fe(NO_3)_3 + 3 NO_2 + 3 H_2O$$

Highly Conc. and pure HNO_3 makes it passive.

iv) With dil and conc. HCl forms hydrogen and Ferrous chloride.

$$2 HCl + Fe \text{------------------} FeCl_2 + H_2 \text{ (Ferrous chloride)}$$

v) With dil H_2SO_4 forms ferrous sulphate and hydrogen.

$$Fe + H_2 SO_4 \text{------------------} Fe SO_4 + H_2$$

With Conc. H_2SO_4 gives a mixture of ferrous sulphate, ferric sulphate and sulphur dioxide.

$$2 H_2SO_4 + Fe \text{--------------} Fe SO_4 + SO_2 + 2 H_2O$$

$$2 Fe SO_4 + 2 H_2SO_4 \text{---------------} Fe_2(SO_4)_3 + 2 H_2O + SO_2$$

vi) With copper sulphate forms ferrous sulphate and metallic copper is precipitated.

$$Fe + Cu SO_4 \text{------------------} Fe SO_4 + Cu \downarrow$$

Comparison of Cast Iron, Wrought Iron and Steel are given in the tabular form:

Property	Cast Iron	Wrought Iron	Steel
1. Composition	From 94-96% carbon 2-5% impurities (P, Si, S, Mn)-1.5%	From 98.5-98.8% Carbon 0-2-0.5% impurities-1%	From 98.5-99.5 Carbon 0.5-1.5%
2. Hardness	Hard	Soft	Medium Hardness
3. Brittleness	Brittle	Malleable	Malleable and brittle depending upon conditions
4. Magnetic Properties	Cannot be permanently magnetised	Magnetisation is not permanent	Can be permanently magnetised
5. Tempering	Cannot be tempered	Cannot be tempered	Can be tempered
6. Welding	Can't be welded	Can be welded	Can be welded

QUESTIONS

1. a) Describe the extraction of iron from its principal ores, giving a neat sketch of the furnace used and the probable reactions occuring there in.

    b) Write notes on the following: i) Tempering of steel. ii) Nitriding of steel.   (W - 1988)

2. a) What do you understand by the term "heat treatment"? Discuss the various types of heat treatment of steel.

    b) Compare open hearth process with Bessemer process for the manufacture of steel.

    c) Complete the following equations and rewrite the equation, naming the products formed.

i)   Fe + Steam --------------------

ii)   Fe + hot and conc. sulphuric acid --------------------

iii) Fe + cold and dil. nitric acid ----------------------

iv)   Fe + strong nitric acid --------------------

v)   Fe + copper sulphate ----------------------   (S-1989)

3. a) Name any two ores of Iron.

    b) Draw a neat and labbled diagram of the blast furnace used in extraction of Iron.

    c) Give the chemical reactions which take place at different stages.   (W-1989)

4. a) Name the important ore of aluminium.

    b) Describe the process involved in the extraction of pure aluminium metal from its ore.

5. a) Name any two ores of Iron.

    b) How is wrought Iron manufactured?

    c) Compare and contrast the properties of cast iron, wrought iron and steel.   (S-1990)

6. a) Describe the extraction of iron from its principal ores giving a neat sketch of the furnace used and the possible reactions occuring there in.

    b) Write notes on the following:

i) Tempering ii) Nitriding.

c) What is the action of the following on iron.

i) Air ii) Steam iii) Dil sulphuric acid iv) Hot and conc. sulphuric acid. v) copper sulphate. (S-1988)

7. Choose and rewrite the correct answers to the following:

i) Better quality of steel is obtained by

a) Bessemer process. b) Open hearth process.

ii) Haematite is concentrated by

a) Gravity separation b) Forth floatation process c) Electromagnetic process

iii) Carbon content is maximum in

a) Cast Iron b) Wrought Iron c) Steel

iv) Permanent magnets can be made from

a) Cast iron b) Wrought Iron c) Steel

v) In the open hearth process for the manufacture of steel fuel used is:

a) Producer gas b) oil gas c) coal gas (W-1988)

8. *Fill in the blanks:*

i) The melting point of an alloy is -------------- than that of pure metals

ii) An alloy is a homogenous ----------- of metal-metal.

iii) Object of alloy making is to improve its -----------.

iv) Stainless steel is ---------- by magnet.

v) Stainless steel is ---------- to corrosion. (S-1988)

9. a) Describe the different methods used for refining.

b) Explain the following terms: i) Flux ii) Smelting iii) Cupellation iv) Slag ·v) Gangue. (W-1988)

10.a) Describe briefly the principal steps employed for the extraction of metals from their ores.

Illustrate each step by example.

b) Differentiate the following with suitable examples;

      i) Roasting and Calcination.

      ii) Flux and Slag.

      iii) Ore and Mineral.

c) Write notes on the following;

      i) Types of Metallergy.

      ii) Electrolytic refining.   (S-1989)

11.a) Explain the following terms:

      i) Flux ii) Slag iii) Gangue.

b) Describe the following.

      i) Roasting ii) Smelting.

c) Write note on Electro refining.   (W-1989)

12.a) What is difference between a mineral and ore.

b) Explain the following terms (any three)

   (1) Flux (2) Smelting (3) Cupellation. (4) Froth-floation process (5) Electro refining.

c) Complete the following statements:

      i) Sulphide Ores are usually concentrated ------------------.

      ii) Copper is concentrated by -------------------.

      iii) Heating of the ore in the presence of air is called ----------.

      iv) Carbonate ores are usually subjected to ------------------.

v) Smelting is usually done ------------------ furnace. (S-1990)

13.a) Describe the different methods used for refining.

b) Outline the methods used for extraction of metals.

c) Complete the following:

      i) The process of removing earthy impurities from the ore is known as --------------.

      ii) Slag is lighter then the ------------------.

      iii) In the froth floatation process the powdered Ore is agitated with a mixture of -------------------.

    iv) Oxide Ores are generally concentrated by ----------------.

    v) Flux is a substance used to remove in fusible impurities in the form of --------------   (S-1988)

ANSWERS:

2.   c) i) $3 Fe + 4 H_2O$ --------------- $Fe_3O_4 + 4 H_2$

      Products: ferroso Ferric oxide and Hydrogen.

    ii) $Fe + 2 H_2SO_4$ ------------ $Fe SO_4 + SO_2 + 2 H_2O$

       $2 Fe SO_4 + 2 H_2SO_4$ ---------- $Fe_2 (SO_4)_3 + 2 H_2O + SO_2$

      Products: a mixture of ferrous sulphate, ferric sulphate, sulphur dioxide and water.

    iii) $4 Fe + 10 HNO_3$ ----------- $4 Fe (NO_3)_2 + NH_4NO_3 + 3H_2O$

      Products: Ferrous nitrate, ammonium nitrate and water.

    iv) $Fe + 6 HNO_3$ ------------ $Fe (NO_3)_3 + 2 NO_2 + 3 H_2O$

      Fairly strong.

      Products: Ferric nitrate, nitrogen peroxide and water.

      Highly conc. and pure HNO_3 makes it passive

    v) $Fe + Cu SO_4$ ---------------- $Fe SO_4 + Cu$

      Products: Ferrous sulphate and metallic copper is precipitated.

7.   i- (b) ii- (a) iii- (a) iv- (c) v- (a)

8.   i) Lower ii) mixture iii) properties iv) not attracted v) resistant.

12.c   i) Froth floatation process.
     ii) -do- in the case of Sulphide Ores.
     iii) Oxidation.
     iv) Calcination.
     v) Reverberatory.

13.c   i) Concentration.
     ii) Metal
     iii) Water and pine oil.
     iv) Washing.
     v) Slag.

PHONES: 3276712
3271632

CBS PUBLISHERS AND DISTRIBUTORS
11, DARYA GANJ, ANSARI ROAD NEW DELHI-110002

RECEIVED/SEND COMPLIMENTARY Copy/Copies of

_____

_____

_____

_____

SIGNATURE_____

SEAL

DESIGNATION_____

DATE _____

COLLEGE/SCHOOL_____

ADDRESS_____

FULL NAME_____

HOME ADDRESS_____

_____

Signature of Representative